Friday's Child

Friday's Child

THE THREAT TO MORAL EDUCATION

by

Carol Lee

To Meryl o all at Hen-Blas, With love from Carol.

THORSONS PUBLISHING GROUP

First published 1988

© Carol Lee 1988

British Library Cataloguing in Publication Data

Lee Carol
 Friday's child: the threat to moral
 education
 1. Sex instruction for children—Great
 Britain
 I. Title
 613.9'5'071041   HQ53

 IBSN 0-7225-1449-2

Published by Thorsons Publishers Limited,
Wellingborough, Northamptonshire, NN8 2RQ, England

Printed in Great Britain by Biddles Limited, Guildford, Surrey

10 9 8 7 6 5 4 3 2 1

Contents

Acknowledgements

I would like to thank all the people who have continued to support this work, especially Derek Steward, headmaster of Chase Cross School, Romford, Essex and Martin Hayes, the head of sixth year. I would also like to thank Tony Selina for editing this book so sensitively and Jackie Glass for encouraging me to persevere with it.

Introduction

'*It is essential that attitudes to sex are taught in a clearly moral framework.*' Peter Bruinvels (when an MP), Education Bill, Hansard, October 1986.

'*Teaching about the physical aspects of sexual behaviour should be set within a clear moral framework...*' Department of Education and Science Circular No 11/87, 25 September, 1987.

The people who are against sex education used to argue that it shouldn't be taught at all. When this position (which I referred to as 'The Ostrich Position') became publicly unacceptable the argument shifted to talk of morals. This was a clever move since it is difficult to get two concerned people to agree completely on any moral point of view, let alone one connected with sex education, the role of parents and the development of teenagers. There is no fixed consensus on these moral issues. Hence 20 school governors could spend years discussing what 'a moral framework' is and whether it hinders or serves learning as they understand it. By this time the subject will have disappeared from the school curriculum — and this is what has been happening.

Many times during the course of teaching sex education I have been divided about whether to spend more time in the classroom doing this work or on public platforms protecting it. My preference was for the former but as it happens the decision was taken away from me by attacks on sex education from a group of people I have called the Moral Right.

The morality of education in general and of sex education in particular, and of the people who oppose these issues as I understand them, is something I have set out to explore in this book. As before it has been with the help of teenagers, and it is therefore in the classroom that I shall begin, for the moral issues that one faces in working with pupils are not what the Moral Right would have us — or themselves — believe.

Dedication

To the pupils, once more, with my thanks for their honesty, patience and enthusiasm.

CHAPTER ONE

We love you but...

The classroom is a strange place when you think about it. More often than not it is a room designed with little regard for human efficiency, aesthetics, or for anything else except containment. In it are gathered 20 to 30 young people who did not know each other before going to secondary school. They are also strangers to Her Majesty's Government, which detains them by compulsory order, as sanctioned in the Education Acts. They are in school to be taught 'subjects' by a specialist called a teacher. Everyone in the classroom is there to work (although only the teacher is paid for this), and in some cases the work is not made easy.

I never thought to describe schooling like this until I walked into a classroom one day a few years ago as a visiting teacher. It was winter, or at least November — one of those grey, bleak days when it is difficult to want to do anything else but huddle by a fire. The school playground looked particularly stark; a small patch of uneven concrete, windy and deserted. What seemed like a watchman, though he was no doubt a caretaker, directed me up rows of cold stone steps through chilly, dingy corridors to a reception office a few flights up. In here, at least, the picture was different — startlingly so. Three women worked in a pleasant if somewhat overcrowded office with large windows giving a view over the city. The room was light and warm and felt friendly. I waited for ten minutes while they tried to find the teacher whose class I was to take for two weeks for a subject called 'sex education'. It seemed he had forgotten I was coming and was not in the building. Another teacher eventually came and led me through a labyrinth of drab corridors to a classroom on the ground floor. By the time we got there I was 15 minutes late for a session lasting one hour and ten minutes. The teacher had said practically noth-ing as we hurried through the inhospitable maze. Now he called the straggled class to order and said 'Miss Lee has come to talk to you today. Behave yourself, Micky. Sit down and shut up. If

Miss Lee tells me there's been trouble from any of you there'll be some explaining to do afterwards.' With an apologetic look in my direction he headed for the exit. I remembered just in time to say:

'Oh, excuse me. Is there any chalk here?'

'John, come with me', he ordered, and said to me: 'I'll send him back with some'.

It would be exaggerating to say that the classroom was big enough to play football in, but only just. It would not be exaggerating to say that the game would have been impossible to play, not so much for lack of space as for lack of light. The ceiling of the classroom was high. It seemed like a church. The whole place looked grey and lost. Hanging from the high ceiling were strips of light which glared in places and cast shadows in others. The school had high walls, with windows near the top, the kind the Victorians built to stop pupils from breaking windows — or from climbing out. Certainly the urge to escape from a place like this would be strong in any healthy, normal person. The place reminded me of something, and sitting in the car afterwards I remembered what it was. I had once interviewed a Chilean actress about her time as a prisoner in the infamous Santiago gaol where unspeakable tortures were carried out on her and many others. She had vividly described to me her time there and in particular the room where she was first taken. I hadn't thought to question it at the time, but she had described this room as being 'like a classroom' with a large blackboard at one end in a high-ceilinged, bare room with strip-lighting giving it a strange harshness and bleakness at the same time. There were rows of tables in the room and a man in military dress was standing near the blackboard, some documents in his hand.

This was like the venue for today's work.

'Okay,' I said, as John came hurrying back and about 15 faces looked towards me — in some anticipation by this time. 'We'd better begin. First of all I would like to apologize to you all for being so late...' I paused and realized that practically everyone in the room was wearing a coat, as I still was. 'Are most of you cold?' I asked. There was a moment's silence and then someone said:

'It's nearly always cold in here, Miss.'

I looked around for the nearest radiator, and walking over to it discovered that it was slightly warm.

'A lot of this session has gone by in any case', I said, 'so a few minutes won't make much difference. Would you all please gather round these tables near the radiator. It might be easier to work if we don't have our coats on.'

The atmosphere in the room at this stage was extremely low-key. The pupils moved listlessly and I really wasn't sure how to begin the work called 'education' in such muted surroundings. So I began something like this: 'Why do you think I'm here today? What do you think we're going to talk about, or learn? And is this different from what you would like to talk about or learn?' There was an awkward silence. I had asked too much at once. But at least we'd started, so I repeated: 'Why do you think I'm here? What kind of issues and topics are we going to talk about?'

A girl said 'Abortion, Miss.'

I waited. A boy said 'Contraception and things like that.'

'Anything else?' I said.

'Feelings,' a boy said flatly as if he'd learned it parrot-fashion and was repeating to me something he thought I wanted to hear, rather than what he himself wanted to say or know. But he'd given me a way in.

'I want to know what you all feel about this room,' I said. They looked at each other in disbelief and a mixture of boredom and consternation. 'After that I want to know something else from you,' I added, to try and awaken their interest, 'but for the present let's stick with this room. Come on, I'll begin. This room makes me feel flat and unenergetic.'

'It's just a room,' one girl ventured defensively.

No more.

'You're not with me', I said, 'so let's go quickly from person to person round the class. We've got to waken up in here. I want each of you tell me quickly in a sentence or two about a room, any room, you enjoy. I nodded to a boy on my left, who hesitated and then said: 'I like my bedroom because it's got all my own things in it and it's small and it feels safe.' He looked a bit embarrassed at the last bit, but I nodded seriously and we went round in just a few minutes with everyone describing their own or their shared bedroom. I noted privately that their need for safety and privacy, away from this classroom — and me — was strong. But they had begun to wake up, especially since, at the end, as I usually do in these round robin exchanges, I gave my own contribution. I described my living room and they obviously responded to my description of its warmth and homeliness. So we began from here to discuss how feelings can be altered by our surroundings and how we can respond the other way round and have our feelings transcend surroundings so that we forget about them if they're unpleasant. We talked about being 'in love' as an instance of this. We were deep into this discussion when one girl said suddenly:

'But it isn't only this room, Miss. There's something else...' She hesitated and a boy hissed at her:

'Shut up, you berk.'

'Please let her speak now that she's begun,' I asked him, and the girl, with some misgivings, explained. It wasn't only the room that was making them feel bad that morning. At the moment a boy called Tom, who was usually with them, was lying seriously ill in hospital after trying to commit suicide.

'Only we're not supposed to know that, Miss.'

'How *do* you know?', I asked.

Another girl said: 'Because my mum went round to his house, not knowing it had happened and his mum told her and she told me.'

'She shouldn't have done that,' someone else said.

'Why not?' I asked.

'Because it's upsetting,' a girl replied.

This left me in a terrible quandary, and as they all looked at me expectantly my mind was racing furiously. Since Tom was in hospital I had to be very careful not to talk about him in any way that would further alienate him from this group of people, who would be important to his recovery — presuming that he did recover. At the same time I couldn't just ignore what they'd told me. It mattered to them and they obviously had strong feelings about it, and their having told me was their way of saying that they needed help with it. In all this I had to act cautiously. So I started slowly: 'I'm grateful to you', I said to the girl, 'for confiding in me, and to all of you for letting me know this.' I paused. 'The problem we have to work out is what it is best to do, and we'll have to work this out together.'

We were all extremely attentive at this point. I was moving slowly, thinking out loud in order to let them know what I was doing, and to give myself more time to work out a way of discussing their feelings without talking about Tom behind his back. Eventually I hit on what I thought was a compromise and said: 'I think we all *should* talk about this, and as long as we are careful there will be no harm done.' I suggested to them that I thought we should all write down on paper some of the feelings and thoughts about what Tom had done — myself included. We would have to be extremely careful not to discuss the boy himself or make comments about his actions. Since we were the people who were here we should discuss ourselves and our own feelings about an event, not the event itself. I illustrated this for them with the following two sentences: 'My friend was mean to me because she didn't invite me to her birthday party,' and 'I feel hurt and left out because I would have liked to have gone to a birthday party.' I said that after we had all written our feelings down on bits of paper, without putting our names on them, I would jumble up the bits of paper and read them to all of us. They looked a bit shocked at this so I said: 'It's important to do this, and it's also important therefore that you only write down what you want to share safely. I assure you that you will be able to tell me afterwards why I insisted on reading out all the bits of paper and not just some of them.' I asked them if they wanted to do this.

'We know what you mean', said one boy, 'about not talking about Tom when he's not here, but that's all we've been thinking about and sometimes we've shouted at each other for talking about it.'

'Okay', I said, 'let's do as I suggest. I want you to write at least 50 words or three medium-sized sentences. You may say what you like as long as you are happy to do this and don't want to keep some feelings to yourself. You may be as angry as you like, or as cool as you like. If this hasn't affected you, or you are irritated by all the fuss, then say that too. I want you to write this in silence, as I will, unless there's a question you want to ask or some help you need. I'll give you about ten minutes.'

The whole atmosphere had been highly emotionally charged ten minutes earlier and I'm sure we had all completely forgotten what room we were in. I certainly had. Now the energy had levelled down to one of those rare atmospheres which I can only describe as a kind of contentment. This is particularly uncommon in a secondary school. I've often come across it in primary schools where children are so much more open to learning and where you see 20 heads bent down in one common cause, perhaps trying to write their day's diary. This kind of shared concentration and enterprise is one that I value and it's to our detriment that we don't continue it, in part, into secondary schools and adult life, for it is possible to do so given some thought and effort. It reminds us that we *do* have a common bond, that we can be co-operative and that they rewards from this are what this group afterwards described as 'good feelings'. My own good feelings that day came from looking round me and seeing the different expressions on people's faces as they applied themselves to what was both a separate and a common task, and my own satisfaction as I bent my head to join them.

I began writing my own contribution carefully because while I had to be honest I also had to be wary. I didn't want to leave them with something that could be disturbing. After waiting for everyone to finish they passed their folded bits of paper along the desk and I jumbled them up and started reading them. One had written 'It's wrong to commit suicide, and before we started talking about it I just thought that. I didn't have sympathy because it's a stupid thing to do, and my mum says it's wicked. Now I feel confused about it. I don't want to say any more. I want to know what other people say about it.' Another wrote: 'He was my mate and I'm really angry with him. What a stupid thing to do. I feel really hurt he didn't say. I haven't been to see him in hospital. His mum asked me to go but I couldn't. It won't be the same after this. I know it won't.' He had heavily scored out the last two words, 'Something's died,' and I didn't read them out.

At this stage the school bell rang for the lunch hour. The door opened and the staff member who had brought me in came to take me away again. Yet no-one around me had moved and it was a very bad time indeed to break off and just leave. So I said: 'I'm prepared to stay on for half an hour and finish what we've begun. Do you want me to?' There were nods and murmurs of assent, so I told the teacher I would stay on a bit and then find my own way to the staff room afterwards to have a chat with him. He looked ill at ease and nonplussed, but he left and we resumed work. I continued to read all the bits of paper, making a note as I went along of some of the important points raised. For a start it was obvious that they hadn't managed to leave Tom out of it, but this wasn't surprising. At least they'd tried. It was easy to spot in the main which items were written by girls and which by boys, and this reflected both the fact that Tom was a boy and the fact that, generally, the girls seemed less disturbed by what had happened. I imagined this was mainly because the girls had less difficulty than the boys in understanding the emotional depths which could drive people to such drastic actions. But time was racing by and there were a few important things to cover so as not to leave them with a sense of unfinished business. So I asked: 'At the beginning of the lesson I told you that you would begin to understand why I insisted on reading out all the bits of paper. Do you understand now why I did that?' They thought about this for a moment and a girl asked, rather than answered:

'So we know how each other feels?'

'Yes,' I said, 'and why is that important? Or let's put it another way. Is that important?'

'Yes it is,' said a boy, 'because what people's feelings are matters...'

'And', said another boy, 'if you know how people feel then you know how to treat them.'

'Do you?' I said with a smile. 'In that case we have all learned a great deal today.' I was just about to go on to make a few final points when a girl said:

'Aren't you going to read us your feelings, Miss?'

I'd forgotten about my own piece of paper. I had written: 'I am *pleased* you told me what was troubling you because if you hadn't we wouldn't have learned what we have today. I am *worried* that we have a lot of work to get through in such a short time. I feel *sad* that life is extremely hard for many people. I feel *hope* as well, that by working together we can help make life better for ourselves and for others.' They would have been happy to go right on discussing the points raised here, but I had to call a halt. We had all worked long enough and there could have been people in the group who hadn't yet eaten anything that day. I said at the end that the reason Tom had tried to commit suicide was very much his own business and that I hoped they would all respect this, and that it was *this* they should avoid gossiping about. However, a further discussion of their *own* feelings among each other would be fine if that was what they wanted. I thanked them for staying behind and said I would reserve five minutes at the beginning of the next session in case there was anything more on this they wanted to talk about. I said I wanted to get into talking about relationships and sexuality, and that the work we had done today would make that much easier to do. I asked if someone would show me the way to the staff room and told them all to get something to eat before it was too late.

The staff room was uncarpeted, scruffy and physically drab and depressing, although there was a friendly buzz humming round it. I spotted the staff member I wanted who viewed my approach uneasily. He had already decided there was something about me he would rather not face. While I told him briefly about what had gone on in the classroom he looked around anxiously for a means of escape. Yes, he had heard about the boy's suicide attempt, but no, he didn't know what had been said to the class as a whole. Of course he would look into it with the form teacher concerned. With great relief he suddenly remembered something he had to do and, with ill-concealed haste, departed.

The following week I arrived particularly early and was able to start work on time. It was a markedly different day and bright autumn sun was managing to find its way into parts of the room.

Tom was out of hospital and would soon be back in school. The class was in good spirits, full of energy and very anxious not to waste any time, so I moved quickly. Usually I get pupils to make connections themselves by asking them questions, but this was one of those rare occasions when I felt happy to make some of the connections myself because they were eager to listen. One of the connections I made for them was to state, from the previous week, that the feelings I had written down on my paper were both positive and negative, and that this showed how it was possible for a wide variety of emotions to be present in any one situation or for any one reason. I asked them to bear this in mind as we began to discuss relationships and sexuality. They did, and we discovered, for example, that the feeling of grief can attend a sexual act, and that joy can be present in something we initially view as painful — the obvious example here being childbirth. Another we found was that sometimes, when someone hurts you, it isn't until that happens that you find you've got friends who care about you as well. I'm afraid we never even managed to get to important topics like contraception, abortion or physiology. What we did instead was to find out that anger is a prevalent human feeling and that it often arises out of hurt, frustration or misunderstanding. We found that, considering how prevalent an emotion it is, there wasn't much room in our lives for dealing with anger safely. But we discussed some of the ways this could be done. We discussed some of the dangers of anger not being accommodated or transformed, and once more we came to see that anger, compassion, fear and hope may all be present more or less at the same time, and that whichever emotion 'wins out' depends on our ability to understand and deal with our circumstances. I suggested that the richness of our emotional lives was a gift, not a burden, and an unending source of possibility for change and growth. We went on from there to find out that one of the reasons this did not often seem the case to teenagers was because they felt *at the mercy* of their emotions. They felt particularly at the mercy of the many conflicting emotions which arose in them because of having to accommodate their sexual development, and all that this entails.

We then looked at the subject of 'work'. They discovered, much to their surprise, that we all had worked very hard the previous week, and that as this session drew to a close, had worked even harder this week. Partly they understood this, and partly they didn't. It hadn't felt like work, they said, because it had been easy. Yet I described to them how they had concentrated, as I had, and how they had joined together thoughts, feelings and ideas, and accomplished a tremendous amount in only a few hours. We ended up, more or less, with a round robin again where I asked them each to take it in turn to say a sentence or two about duty. I asked each of them to say what his or her duty was. They said things like: 'It is my duty to be kind,' 'It is my duty to be concerned about others,' and, to much laughter, 'It is my duty to get up in the morning'. But eventually someone got the point: 'It's my duty to understand myself,' he said.

'And if you do that, what will it do for others?' I asked.

'It will help me to understand them as well,' he replied.

It's not often you *ever* reach this point, let alone find you've arrived at it after less than three hours' work. But it was the end of this particular journey. It was time to part company and I thanked them and wished them well. They hovered round as the hooter went, as if they wanted more, as if they didn't want to stop when we had really only just started. On the occasions when this happens I feel very torn. How can one undertake such important work with a group of people and then just walk away leaving them, and yourself, flat? All I could say was: 'It's been lovely working with you, but I have to go. Remember that the work has only just begun.'

As I turned to leave, a few pupils came forward and awkwardly gave me a piece of paper. I was just about to open it when the teacher from the previous week appeared at the door. It was obvious from his demeanour that he had spent the last week wondering how to cope with me, and had come to a firm decision.

'Right,' he said loudly, 'I want all those chairs back where they came from and...' He turned to me. 'I'll show you the way out,' he said and politely steered me towards the door. I stuck the piece of paper in my pocket, and with a smile towards the pupils, left. I walked to the car and opened the piece of paper. On it was hastily written: 'Thank you, Miss, you've helped us. We won't forget it.' The message made me cry.

Funny places, classrooms.

These young people were 14 and 15 years old. Our discussion of emotions and personal relationships shows what level of maturity is possible when young people are allowed what should be theirs: their own quest for personal values. People who demand that teenagers have morality imposed on them as if they were flat packages and we were stamping machines are, as far as I'm concerned, themselves behaving immorally, for their imposed morality tends to stunt individual growth. It also tends to stunt public awareness, for the work I have just described took place against increasingly successful pressure to have it stopped. Although I cannot imagine anyone would object to what took place in those two sessions, there was mounting antagonism towards the context within which it took place: 'sex education'. The pressures against sex education and against young people being allowed to come to terms, through knowledge, with their own bodies and their sexuality, have been overwhelming. Many years ago the argument was that young people shouldn't know about sexuality at all. When it became patently absurd that the facts and feelings of adolescence should be *kept* from adolescents the ground shifted to talk about morals. The opponents of sex education then said it had to be taught within a 'moral framework', or what I would call an 'immoral cage'. This was an excellent smokescreen, since the whole area of morals, let alone the morality of sex education, is so intricate, so prone to cultural differences, and is so value-laden, etc. In the months and years it takes adults to argue about all this, a whole generation of children will grow up behind our backs. The moral lessons to be learned from the whole episode surrounding a boy's attempted suicide, as it affected the young people I worked with, reflect badly on the adults concerned, not on the young people. For example I think it morally reprehensible that no-one at the school had taken the class aside as a group and given them the time to talk about this, if for no better reason than that it was obviously a distraction to them and affected their ability to work. I also find that this illustrates the difference between how we view primary and secondary schools — another thing which is morally perturbing. It's as if we banish children at the age of 11 from a state of innocence called primary school where they learn by being engaged and absorbed, and we forcibly eject them from this educational Garden of Eden into forced labour camps called secondary schools. It's as if the age of 11 marks the difference between the privilege and bliss of childhood, which in part we revere, and apprenticeship for the real adult world which is a wicked and difficult place. It's also interesting that the age of 11 is for many the onset of puberty, the beginning of full or adult sexuality. So are secondary children pulled into line for the fact that they will soon become sexually mature? Surely not. In primary school you have a classroom and a teacher of your own. In secondary school you become squatters in strange rooms where other people also learn, and reluctant nomads in vast corridor networks designed, you would imagine from their perversity of layout, by closet catacomb builders. I find it odd that people who think it was terrible for 8-year-olds to sweep chimneys are pleased for 11-year-olds to be imprisoned by law in some of the secondary schools I have been in. The point is that some secondary schools treat children like unskilled workers. An 11-year-old is taken from the gaily coloured, intimate surroundings of a primary school into the vast network of a secondary school and suddenly told: 'The game's up. No more nice Miss or cosy Sir to mop up your tears. This is business.' One of the things that happens here is that the child goes from the personal to the impersonal, from belonging to alienation, as if childhood is about the former and adulthood about the latter. The 9-year-old decorated her primary school herself and now she is in a place which doesn't belong to her. The moral messages delivered here are extremely perplexing, especially where they relate to maturity and to work. The secondary school as I have so often seen it arranged would have you believe that both work and adulthood are nasty. That message might just as well be written up on the school walls, for I can't believe that a group of 10-year-olds would have been treated with the same callousness as the group of 14- and 15-year-olds I have just described. If this kind of treatment is part of the assault course for maturity then it's no wonder so many people don't make it.

There was a time in the late seventies when sex education was beginning to be more generally accepted. It had begun in the 1950s and 1960s as a response to the need for information on contraception, abortion and VD. Schools at that time had begun to bring in doctors or health visitors to give information on these topics. Some schools approached the Family Planning Association (FPA) for help because of its expertise in the area of contraception. Eventually in the early 1970s the FPA set up an education unit to train a small band of people called 'sex educators', not just in information-giving but in working with young people in sympathetic and educative ways. I was one of a small band who took on work in schools which asked for it. Most schools did not, however, and the teaching was mainly confined to London and a few other large cities like Birmingham and Glasgow. Even so, because the number of people trained was so small, there was still difficulty for a while in meeting demand. This tailed off eventually as schools began to realize that it would be better if their own staff did the work. Again the FPA co-operated by organizing courses for teachers, and stopped training people like me. Due to pressure from the Conservative government the FPA was then asked to give assurances that it would no longer send people like me into schools. As a result I began to teach on a completely freelance basis and am now one of no more than a handful of people doing this.

The political pressure against sex education has continued and because of it the work is now diminishing sharply. This pressure began in earnest with Mrs Gillick's campaign which started in January 1981 and was the first of many to reverse the growing trend towards sex education. because of this I have seen schools move in the last dozen years from beginning this subject with difficulty to accepting it and then backing away from it again under the linked threats of political pressure and financial cutbacks. At the same time I have seen parents move firmly towards wanting schools to take on this subject. In fact most of the parents I now speak with believe that schools do have proper programmes of sex education and that their children are learning both the elementary 'facts of life' and about issues like AIDS, contraception and sexual responsibility, in the classroom. Many parents have tacitly handed over this duty to the schools with relief. The schools which have not capitulated to certain pressures and have continued this work have therefore gone from strength to strength. They have provided pupils with a curriculum, and the staff to match it, where sexuality is viewed as a normal part of development and accepted both generally and specifically into school life. These schools have been able to do this because they have had considerable parental backing and in times of difficulty they have been able to call on this either privately or publicly. As one parent whose son attends such a school said:

> Of course I want to be involved too, but in a different way. I see my role as being to provide a background environment of love, and the school's role to be tackling issues, most of which quite frankly I don't have enough knowledge to tackle myself. I've never had to complain about anything which my son has been taught in this school. I trust the staff, and the Head, and if there were any problems I'm sure my son would tell me about them and we'd sort them out.

What has happened over the years is that the gap between the schools who have taken on the subject and the schools which haven't, or who have faltered, has widened. So although more schools now have sex education as an integral part of education generally, many have fallen behind. And while available research shows us that the vast majority of parents want schools to take on sex education, most schools still do not have programmes for it or plans for its incorporation, and tens of thousands of children are being brought up with hardly any information at all. This is an era where AIDS kills, where unemployment takes its toll on the very heart of being human and where therefore it is even more important to have the abilities and the information to form sustaining relationships. In fact for many young people relationships will be all that they have to sustain them, and while in some ways this is everything if these are good, it is also true that the qualities needed to find, form and keep these relationships need all the more attention and nurturing. Thus self-knowledge, self-esteem, compassion, discernment, toughness where necessary, and the ability to develop inner resources are all as crucial now as they always have been. And it is by ignoring the development of these qualities in the past that many of our present perils have come about.

One of these present perils is the grouping of people I call the Moral Right, who are trying to stop sex education. They are doing so by getting up on a moral platform from which they presume to tell us that their own standards of morality and decency are the only correct ones. They imply that the rest of us are, by deliberation or default, immoral and indecent, particularly if we have the temerity to disagree with them. What they have done, as if of right, is to populate like early Puritan settlers the territory which is called decent common ground. They have taken upon themselves the role of watchdogs of decent standards, guardians of family life and keepers of the nation's morals. These people are both pessimists, for they believe we cannot do this for ourselves, and gaolers, for by setting themselves up as having the key to the issues of morality and decency they deny us our own individual freedom. At a conference I chaired on 'The Family and Morality', journalist and author Jill Tweedie startled and delighted an audience at London's City University when she said that one of the largest threats to the present-day family was the 'expert'. She explained that in presuming to dictate to parents what their children needed, 'experts' very often took away from ordinary folk the common knowledge which we have or would find if only experts would leave us alone to do so. The link here with the Moral Right is to do with interference. Experts are extremely valuable in making available to us the results of their research, but we must then be left to make up our own minds, for what we do know is that experts can be wrong and that leading experts in the same field can vehemently disagree with each other. The Gillick campaign exemplified this.

It is of fundamental importance that people have both the right and the ability to think for themselves. In education at least, *true* morality begins in the assumption that a person is both unique and has therefore a mind of his or her own, and is also a social being with the need to develop the skills and awareness which 'belonging' requires. Looked at from this point of view the setting up of a moral code by one group of people as the only correct one is a problem. As well as taking away from the individual the need and therefore the responsibility for self-determination, it also inhibits its own necessary development by denying itself the change and growth which came about when people are active and critical. Approached in a different way these problems could be avoided. I have no objection to anyone saying, for example, that family life has proved necessary and sustaining to billions of people over the centuries and that it has many essential and valuable attributes. Neither can I object to anyone saying that he or she personally finds family life wonderful. The danger lies in saying that family life of a certain kind is the *only* kind of relationship that is correct, and that all others are wrong.

The group of people I call the Moral Right do make pronouncements of this kind, and seek to impose morality rather than elicit it. At one time this earned them the title 'The Moral Majority', for it was presumed that they spoke for the majority of middle-of-the-road, law-abiding people whose ethics were based soundly on common sense and on living decent, ordinary lives. In other words, most of us. But the Moral Right does *not* speak for the majority of decent people. In fact it has excesses and dangerous flaws which people who care about ethics will travel a long way to avoid.

In general parents are now most concerned that sex education in schools should continue. For parents *have* become more involved in finding out what goes on in schools, and in forming those invaluable links between school and home which benefit everyone, particularly children. However, there was one parent whose public intercession turned back the clock of progress far more than any of us fully bargained for.

CHAPTER TWO

The numbers game

For ten months between January and October 1985 I was 'banned' from going into classrooms to work with pupils who were under the age of 16. I write 'banned' in quotes because no headteacher wrote to me saying: 'you are not allowed'; neither was there a public declaration that I'm aware of, and certainly none involving my own work, which stated: 'Sex education is forbidden to pupils under the age of 16'. If someone had made this kind of statement in public it would have been possible to protest. Effectively, however, it happened without an official word being spoken. It came about because of the considerable efforts of Mrs Victoria Gillick, whose attempts to stop her own daughters from being counselled on certain issues without her consent led her on to a nationwide campaign. In my view the campaign must always have been a nationwide one, for had Mrs Gillick's sole concern been her own children her conduct would necessarily have been different in many important respects. As it was she fought to prevent doctors in particular and certain other professionals working with young people from giving those under 16 years old advice or treatment about sexuality without parental consent. She also fought against a DHSS publication, *Health Service Notice* (80)46, which had in it the following observations:

There is widespread concern about counselling and treatment for children under 16. Special care is needed not to undermine parental responsibility and family stability. The Department would therefore hope that in any case where a doctor or other professional worker is approached by a person under the age of 16 for advice in these matters, the doctor, or other professional, will always seek to persuade the child to involve the parent or guardian (or other person *in loco parentis*) at the earliest state of consultation, and will proceed from the assumption that it would be most unusual to provide advice about contraception without parental consent. It is, however, widely accepted that consultations between doctors and patients are confidential; and the Department recognizes the importance which doctors and patients attach to this principle. It is a principle which applies also to the other professions concerned. To abandon this principle for children under 16 might cause some not to seek professional advice at all. They could then be exposed to the immediate risks of pregnancy and of sexually transmitted disease, as well as other long-term physical, psychological and emotional consequences which are equally a threat to stable family life. This would apply particularly to young people whose parents are, for example, unconcerned, entirely unresponsive, or grossly disturbed. Some of these young people are away from their parents and in the care of local authorities or voluntary organizations standing *in loco parentis*. The Department realizes that in such exceptional cases the nature of any counselling must be a matter for the doctor or other professional worker concerned and that the decision whether or not to prescribe contraception must be for the clinical judgement of the doctor.

Mrs Gillick objected to this. Her eventual response was to commence proceedings which included the statement that:

The said notice has no authority in law and gives advice which is unlawful and wrong, and which adversely affects or may adversely affect the welfare of the plaintiff's said children, and/or the rights of the plaintiff as parent and custodian of the said children, and/or the ability of the plaintiff properly and effectively to discharge her duties as such parent and custodian.

The second part of her declaration went on to say that:

No doctor or other professional person employed... either in the Family Planning Service or otherwise may give any contraceptive and/or abortion advice and/or treatment to any child of the plaintiff below the age of 16 without the prior knowledge and/or consent of the said child's parent or guardian.

An interim judgment in favour of Mrs Gillick came into force on 20 December 1984. This did not of course stop young people being given information, so you could tell a girl under 16 that contraception existed. What you couldn't do was give her guidance about various methods or indeed *give* her contraception itself.

Some doctors took a very liberal view of the difference between information and advice and thereby at least kept in contact with some of their young patients. Others tried to explain the difference to young people. I would have hated to have seen a test case on this, for a 15-year-old would have been torn apart in court for the difference between the two. The verbose wordings and pronouncements of the legal machinery are a mystery to most adults and would certainly confound young people. Is a doctor who tells a 15-year-old that she cannot now have the Pill, but that condoms may be purchased in chemists, 'guilty' of advising or not?

What wasn't appreciated about the interim judgment was that it related not only to doctors. From my own point of view it stopped, wholesale, all the work I was doing with fourth- and some fifth-formers because I work in an exploratory way and not as someone who dishes out information. Had this been appreciated, and had the full wording of the original DHSS Notice been better known about by the public and quoted, for example in the popular press, Mrs Gillick might not have won some of her initial support. Seeing her campaign simply as a mother's attempt to try and make sure that her daughters were not led astray, many people were on her side (although the fact that she named her daughters and not her sons is ethically problematic in itself). It does after all seem a reasonable request to make sure that no-one puts your 15- or even 13-year-old daughter on the Pill without your knowledge. It would also seem reasonable, generally speaking, to discourage very young people from having intercourse, especially in view of AIDS and the increasing number of younger women who are developing pre-cancer of the cervix or who have abnormal smears. So Mrs Gillick could have been viewed as speaking for the decent, middle-of-the-road folk. But that, surely, is what the DHSS circular was doing? What Mrs Gillick was doing was mounting a campaign against under-age sex generally. The issue was something she wanted to bring to, one might almost say impose on, the nation, and as Mrs Gillick has since stated, her family life was in some ways sacrificed to this greater cause both by unwanted public exposure and by individual harrassment of her children. The interchange between Mrs Gillick and her local health authority (West Norfolk and Wisbech) began as a result of the DHSS circular when Mrs Gillick wrote:

> Concerning the new DHSS guidelines on the contraceptive and abortion treatment of children under both the legal and medical age of consent, without the knowledge or consent of the parents, can I please ask you for written assurance that in no circumstances whatsoever will any of my daughters (Beatrice, Hannah, Jessie and Sarah) be given contraceptive or abortion treatment whilst they are under 16, in any of the family planning clinics under your control, without my prior knowledge and irrefutable evidence of my consent? Also, should any of them seek advice in them, can I have your assurance that I would be automatically contacted in the interests of my children's safety and welfare...?

Further letters were exchanged in which West Norfolk and Wisbech were only able to come up with the following: that they would make Mrs Gillick's wishes known to the family planning clinics at Wisbech and King's Lynn and that while the authority accepted the need not to undermine parental responsibility it couldn't give a categorical assurance because 'we believe it is widely accepted that consultations between doctors and patients are confidential and therefore the final decision must be for the doctor's clinical judgement.' In March 1981 Mrs Gillick eventually wrote:

> I formally *forbid* any medical staff employed by Norfolk AHA to give any contraceptive or abortion advice or treatment whatsoever to my four daughters while they are under 16 years, without my consent. Will you please acknowledge this letter and agree whole-heartedly to advise your doctors, etc. to abide by my forbidding.'

Mrs Gillick, one must conclude from this, must have forbidden her daughters to have sex under the age of 16 many times. She must also have felt that they might not obey her, for otherwise taking the matter any further would not have been necessary. In seeking to take her forbidding outside the family Mrs Gillick brought this side of herself to the rest of us, and it says a great deal about our moral disarray (although not in the way Mrs Gillick would look at it) that we let her. One of the major reasons we did so was because of the general success of her wooing of the popular press and the press's use of statistics and figures, many of which were completely inaccurate. In looking back over the large amount of press coverage Mrs Gillick received one becomes startled not only by its volume but by the realization that facts, figures, and indeed quotations were manipulated to an astonishing degree. It would have been almost impossible for any one ordinary person to keep a proper track of what was going on. For example in October 1984 an eminent doctor was quoted in a pro-Gillick article in a national daily as being implicitly against young women being given the Pill. A month later in a different newspaper, this time a regional one, the same doctor was quoted as being angry at the use of his name in this way and described medics who were pro-Gillick as 'irresponsible cranks'. In another leading local paper the previous day another doctor suggested that it was unwise for girls (not women, you will note) to have sex until they were 'at least 20', to prevent cancer of the cervix. Supposedly in support of this, the first doctor was quoted as saying that one in five women under 35 have cervical cancer. In fact he was actually reporting another colleague's findings that out of all women with (all) cancers, one in five was in the under 35 age group — a very different thing altogether. And of the bits I myself have picked up here, are all of them correct, or only one or two, and if so which? Who is to judge? What can be stated quite clearly is that some things can, with effort, be traced back to source, and I have done this in a few examples which follow. Without painstakingly doing this the press cuttings on the Gillick campaign cannot be credible. For instance in another local paper Mrs Valerie Riches, then secretary of the Responsible Society, now Family and Youth Concern, got into the numbers game. She said that the Brook Advisory Centres now found it convenient to say that they saw 2,000 'children' (Mrs Riches' word) a year, but that in a report the previous year they gave the figure as 15,000. Mrs Riches, as reported in the paper, said that if the figure of 15,000 had been wrong Brook should have asked for an apology at the time. As we will see later on Brook may well have done this and got nowhere. Even if they had been completely up to date with all the inaccuracies printed about them, and had had the work-force to deal with each individually, which would have taken some doing, newspapers have ways of printing apologies and corrections where people don't notice them very much. After saying what she had to about Brook, Mrs Riches is then reported as quoting the aforementioned doctor as a testament to her argument, though he had now said in print that he was not on her side. Two recent campaigns have gone a long way towards politicizing the medical profession, which has always tended to be viewed as conservative and certainly on the side of the established order of things. The first was the question of disarmament and the formation of the Medical Campaign Against Nuclear Weapons and the second was Mrs Gillick. Around the early- to mid-eighties it was interesting to see people almost renting doctors to support their stand either for or against Mrs Gillick. Everyone was most anxious to have one. Never were doctors so popular with the physically healthy.

I decided to track down Mrs Riches' figures of 2,000 and 15,000. The DHSS Family Planning Services Form SBL, Summary, July 1984 said: 'The DHSS figures show 600 males and 16,400 females, total 17,000 under-16-year-olds seen at family planning clinics in England in 1983. Of these 173 males and 1,557 females, *total 1,830, were seen at Brook Advisory Centres.*' (My italic.)

Actually, the original figure of 15,000 which Mrs Riches gave is quoted in the Brook Advisory Centre's Annual Report, 1983-84 on page nine and comes in the following sentence: 'Some people are surprised to realize that many more under-16s are seen in family planning clinics (15,800, England, 1982) than in Brook where 2,100 clients were under 16 this year'. At about the same time as I was wading through the files on Mrs Gillick I was also trying to find out for a TV programme I was taking part in how many women died of cancer of the cervix in Britain in 1986. In a period covering seven weeks the figures given for 1985-86 varied from 568 to 2,100 — in other words by a factor of more than three. So the problem of the reporting of figures would seem to be a general one.

The numbers game is certainly a problem in itself, as were some of the stories that were put out during the Gillick campaign — some cynically and some not. There were the predictable comments such as the ones which described the Pill being doled out to children like sweets, and then the stories about Muslim girls being shocked by explicit sex education. What was certainly always predictable was that the stories nearly always concerned girls. It was as if boys did not have a part to play in this moral spectrum called under-age sex, and in its consequences. As for the figures themselves, on the one hand the Brook Advisory Centres told us that teenage pregnancies were falling and on the other Family and Youth Concern told us they were rising drastically. On the one hand DHSS figures told us teenage abortions had levelled off, on the other hand a doctor speaking from the Moral Right told us these figures had reached the level of a national scandal. In November 1984 one health authority raised a storm by refusing contraceptives to under-16s and a few months later, after a temporary ruling in Mrs Gillick's favour, another raised a storm by refusing to stop giving contraceptives to existing clients who were under 16. On the one side people wrote in to say that here was a woman with important standards which today's society lacked and on the other side people wrote to say she was an interfering meddler. She was called courageous, and then again hopelessly misguided. Petitions were signed for and against her, and no doubt counter-petitions also. It was the figures which were always a problem. Mrs Riches stuck to hers and also claimed that abortions among under 16s were doubling at a time when Brook claimed they were holding steady or falling slightly. Headlines quite literally followed suit and went from 'ABORTIONS UP' to 'ABORTION FIGURES DOWN'. I went to Hansard to look at the figures for myself. Hansard, 22 June 1982, gives a fall in the teenage pregnancy rate for 15-19s and a fall in each year band in that category. Hansard, 21 November 1984, gives a table of figures from

Mr Kenneth Clarke which show that between 1969 and 1982 the number of births in England and Wales to all under-16s dropped, as did the percentage rate of births to those age groups. In 1969 1,236 15-year-olds gave birth and in 1982 that figure was 952. The percentage drop was from 3.82 per thousand girls to 2.42 per thousand. However in 1983 this figure rose to 1,050 and the percentage to 2.92. By this time Mrs Gillick's campaign was well under way. It was stated by Brook that it would give rise to an increase in under-age pregnancies, and at the time the Moral Right said this wasn't exactly the point because girls would not be having sex in the first place if we did not live in a society which condoned such bad practices.

Brook, supposedly the facilitators of such bad things, themselves fell foul of a bad practice of an entirely different hue in late 1983. At the beginning of November a case at the Old Bailey of a man being prosecuted for sex offences against four under-age girls brought forth the *Sun* headline on 5 November: 'JUDGE LASHES OUT OVER GIRL, 10, ON THE PILL'. Counsel had said in court that one of the girls who was then 15 had got the Pill from Brook at the age of 10. Brook has a policy of complete confidentiality towards the people it sees and its then chairperson, Caroline Woodroffe, initially kept confidence. Her files showed that in fact the girl *had* been to Brook and had been given the Pill at the age of 13, which tallied with her present age as given in court. However, since young girls were already scared enough by what was going on generally, Mrs Woodroffe felt it would be wrong to scare any of them further by breaking confidence in this case. And she stuck to this, after seeking advice, until finally on 7 November 1983 the *Standard* had the banner headline: 'WHY WE GAVE PILL TO GIRL OF TEN'.

Mrs Woodroffe circulated a letter to concerned staff members explaining why she had acted as she did:

> 'We immediately decided the only way to stop the story was to tell the press this girl *had* been to us, that she was 13 and that she told us the truth about her age. We did not give any more details about her. It was far too late. The papers went on saying she was 10 right up to the *News of the World* on 13 November. The coincidence with Victoria Gillick's petition was heaven-sent to her cause and the political effects will be long term. If this were to happen again I would refute any such damaging misinformation about Brook immediately, provided that (as in this case) it did not involve adding any information about a client to that already in the press.

Mrs Woodroffe was right in her assessment of the political consequences and she was right partly because of the way the popular press is organized. In it the game is to grab headlines, for it is headlines which sell papers and stick in people's minds, not small print, and certainly not reasoned explanations. So, even if it was, as happened, completely inaccurate, the headlines which talked of 'GIRL, TEN, ON PILL' were the ones that did the damage. While 13 is also very young to be having sexual intercourse, it *is* significantly different from 10. What happened to *young people* as a result of Mrs Gillick's campaign was that they were thrown into confusion. When you realize the amount of confusion adults were in themselves, this is hardly surprising. Clinics reported that girls weren't coming in because they thought they couldn't or because they feared the service was no longer confidential, and I know from my own work in classrooms since the end of 1985 that pupils were very confused about what was and was not possible. When Mrs Gillick won the second stage of her fight in December 1984 she called it a wonderful Christmas present for families and a triumph for parents up and down the land. Five or six weeks later I did a number of interviews which were published in *The Guardian* on Wednesday, 30 January 1985, under the headline VICTORY FOR MRS GILLICK IS A TRAGEDY FOR THOUSANDS OF YOUNG PEOPLE. The article ran as follows:

The young woman doctor was visibly angry. She said: 'I'll go to court if I have to. I'll stake my career on it. I am not going to be ordered to abandon that girl.' The girl in question was 14. She looked 12. She was living alone with her father — and was pregnant by him. The burn marks on her body she would not at first talk about. They were accidents, she said. It took many hours of a counsellor's and doctor's time to learn the truth of her predicament, which is this:

Her father had been having sexual intercourse with her for a year. [Before] that he had manipulated her sexually since the death of her mother, six years previously. When she complained of the pain of intercourse he burned her with matches — to show her what real pain was about. He played games with her where she was offered the match, or sexual intercourse. She chose the latter. She was petrified, and the last thing she wanted was for her father to go to prison.

The doctor said: 'It's fully understandable that she wants to protect her father. Whatever we think of him, in her eyes he is her provider, and also her lover. He is all she has. Is the law of the land telling me I have to go to him to get permission to advise her? I know this is an emergency case, but what happens while we are waiting for the girl to be made a ward of court? She needs our help now. There isn't time to wait.'

The doctor continued: 'I didn't start reading carefully about incest until recently when I came across a report from the London borough of Hackney, which talked of how our knowledge and statistics about incest fall well short of the true picture. A recent American survey showed that in one state alone one in five children had been involved in incest.

'What does the present ruling say about this? What are we supposed to do when a girl of 15 turns up wanting the post-coital (morning-after) pill because her stepfather or an older brother has had intercourse with her? Do we have to ask for parental consent to treat her?'

The problem of incest is one that the high court judgment does not address. Yet in clinics in England and Wales, staff are hearing stories from women, including girls under 16, which show up this particular lie to the notion of 'parental responsibility', to the assumption that these two words automatically go together.

In a London clinic run by the Brook Advisory Centre, another doctor spoke about the case of a young mother who brought in her 15-year-old daughter. The daughter was having a relationship with the mother's ex-lover, a man in his late thirties. The mother wanted her daughter put on the Pill. The girl didn't want this.

The doctor said: 'The three of us went into all the legal aspects, and the mother was not prepared to stop her daughter from continuing with this relationship, but she did want her given contraception.

'We see a number of under-16-year-olds who are brought in by mothers who want them "put on the Pill" when the girls themselves do not want contraception. In some cases the mothers have imagined their daughters are having sexual relationships when in fact the girls are still virgins. In other cases the daughters have had sexual relationships, but have ended them, and have no desire to start others. Are we to follow parental orders here? I certainly do not.

'I am concerned with the client and her overall well-being, and the present ruling means that I am not allowed to act caringly towards clients.

'I am thinking particularly of the young women who have been with us for perhaps a year, whose trust we have gained. Now when they come back to be I am no longer able to continue treating them, unless they gain parental consent. Since our service is based on confidentiality this frightens a lot of girls who imagine that we're now going to tell their parents they have been to us. This is not the case. We still preserve confidentiality, but some girls are running away without understanding this. And they're at risk.'

Health authorities, Brook and other voluntary organization

clinics provided contraception for 17,590 under-16-year-olds in England and Wales in 1983. This represents one in a hundred of client users of all ages.

A clinic secretary in a London borough said: 'The past month here has been absolute chaos. I sometimes go home and cry about what is happening. I feel as if my hands are chained behind my back. I want to help, but I'm not allowed to any more.'

The woman, who is in her late thirties, said: 'We have about 1,000 clients here, with a slightly higher percentage of under-16-year-olds than most clinics. We have spent the last five years gaining the confidence of these girls, telling them not to lie about their ages, educating them about responsibility and about the necessity of being truthful'.

'We make every effort to get under-16s to tell their parents and their GPs, and sometimes, after they have been with us for a while, they do. Parents sometimes thank us for taking care of their daughters. One girl who came to us when she was 14, eventually told her mother a few months ago. Her mother then came in with her and told us what we already knew: how difficult life had been at home for herself and her daughter, until the stepfather left. She was very grateful to us for helping her daughter through this time and for providing her with somewhere to come and talk.

'We're delighted when this happens. But girls need time, and now they haven't got it.

'What is now heartbreaking is that the only way a 15-year-old can be seen without parental consent is if she lies about her age. And they're not doing this. They've got used to trusting us and they come in and tell you they're 14 and 15. Then you have to say you can't treat them. So they're penalised for being truthful.'

'What is particularly worrying is the number of under-16s who have not come back for appointments booked a few months ago. What will happen to them? I had a call from a girl the other day who was almost beside herself with fear. She was ringing to say she wasn't coming back but were we now going to tell her parents she had been to us? I assured her we wouldn't, but it took a long time to persuade her. I had her file in front of me and realized from it that she had a violent father who beat up her mother regularly and who she thought would kill her if he found out she was seeing us. In the middle of our conversation she started sobbing in the call box and begging me not to tell on her.

'I wonder, also, if people realize how sexist this ruling is in real terms. It is young women who are suffering. Young men rarely present themselves for contraception and have other places to go if we can't see them.'

At another family planning clinic the woman who runs it said, grimly: 'I won't tell you what our thoughts about Mrs Gillick have been these last few weeks, except to say that all the staff here have been devastated by the amount of human misery this judgment is causing. It goes without saying that we're all having to work terribly long hours to cope with the deluge of phone calls and visits from badly frightened under-16s who now feel abandoned and terribly confused.

'I don't know how many girls are already pregnant as a result of this ruling. What I do know is that an awful lot of caring, professional people are putting themselves on the line. Like, for example, the head of year at a secondary school who wrote to us last week about a 14-year-old pupil who had been raped. She felt it was impossible, because of the family background, to let the parents know she was sending the girl to us, and she hoped that, despite the judgment, we could help.

'Our present advice is that doctors have to use their own discretion in assessing when post-coital contraception is an emergency, and in this case the doctor in charge dealt with it as such, and prescribed. Our problem now is how to continue seeing this client. The ruling says we cannot give advice, and yet the girl badly needs confidential counselling. She was numb when she arrived here, and unless she is allowed to unlock this experience and really talk about it she will be permanently damaged.

'We have asked her back for counselling, without her parents' permission, for as soon as we mentioned her home the girl just shook her head and started walking out. She is petrified we are going to tell her parents. We won't, but to be honest with you I have no idea whether or not we are within our legal rights in continuing to see her.

'It's really come to something when a teacher, a doctor, a nurse, a counsellor and myself, all professional people, have possibly put ourselves outside the law in order to try to save one young person from a lifetime of misery.

'At the moment doctors feel they are being encouraged, through the plight of young people, to bend the meaning of the word 'emergency'. The present judgment makes an exception of emergency cases and, in the case of post-coital contraception for example, some doctors are saying: 'I shall not stop prescribing this. I shall call in an emergency *per se.*'

Since the 20 December ruling two health authorities have stated openly that they will continue to treat existing under-16-year-old clients for contraception, arguing that it would be a dereliction of duty not to do so. They are, however, not taking on new clients who are under 16 without parental consent.

A family planning nurse said: 'There is no doubt there will be an increase in pregnancies in the under-16-age-group as a result of this ruling. If the ruling is overturned in the House of Lords it will still take many months for clients to begin coming back to us and trusting us again. I even feel it is wrong, for their sakes, to be giving interviews, because it will make them all the more fearful that we don't keep confidence with them.

'It seems, though, that it has to be done. People need to know that what has been a personal victory for Mrs Gillick is a tragedy for thousands of young people and for people, like the staff here, who have spent years building up relationships with clients we are now having to abandon.

'Many young people go through times when they do not want to talk with their parents. Who are they now to turn to?'

Some time after this article was published I was asked to appear on television with Mrs Gillick to discuss her campaign, or should I say to oppose it, for I was invited along with Anna Raeburn to present the 'other' point of view. What was actually strange about this, I now see, was that it was in fact Mrs Gillick who held the 'other' point of view, not us. Both Anna Raeburn and myself held views which concurred, broadly speaking, with the DHSS circular. Yet so firmly entrenched had Mrs Gillick's media campaign become that by 1985 it was assumed that it was *she* who held the majority view and the rest of us — i.e. anyone who opposed her — the 'other' one. I was soon to find out a little of how this media campaign may have been organized. I was asked to arrive at Thames Television early to look at a film called *Let's Talk about Love,* which featured Mrs Valerie Riches. I found it most edifying to watch the film, which gave a black and white version of a tart and a princess. It told of two kinds of girls, those who do and those who don't, one of whom gets the white wedding and one of whom doesn't. I would have found it most useful to show the film in schools to illustrate how morality is not in fact black and white, and also to illustrate some interesting points about the film's intrinsic sexism.

Mrs Gillick, whom I had never met before, came into the green room, which is where people sit while they are waiting to go into television studios. The first thing that struck me about her was her girlish appearance and I was reminded of an article by Anne Robinson in the *Daily Mirror* (9 November, 1983) in which she described Mrs Gillick in the following way: 'She wears Laura Ashley dresses and a remarkable number of small different coloured bows in her hair... Mrs Victoria Gillick might look like a cross between Mary Poppins and the lead part in *The Sound of Music*. But she and her crusade are far more selfish and dangerous than that.'

The second thing which struck me about Mrs Gillick was her temperament. As soon as she heard who I was she became very agitated. She said she would not go on the programme if I did. She shouted and told the producers that they could cancel the programme — they didn't have a programme if I was going on because she wouldn't appear on the same platform as me. As staff came over to apologize to me for this rudeness, and Mrs Gillick was led away to continue her haranguing, the third thing that struck me was what incredible media manipulation this was. Mrs Gillick's name was an audience draw, while mine was not. She could therefore afford to play on this. I wouldn't dare to tell a TV producer who should or should not be on a programme unless I was involved in making it.

In the end, I found myself in the audience, which had been, I think, then producer's original intention anyway. Had it not been, the Mrs Gillick was certainly successful in manipulating the programme to the format in which she wanted it.

The show was something of an ordeal for me and I have been glad to forget most of it (although I do remember a spontaneous round of applause to Anna Raeburn's emotionally charged comment 'I am sick of the Moral Right beating its drum to the detriment of the nation's children'). Afterwards I watched Mrs Gillick with a group of teenage girls of about 16 or 17. I say 'watched' because there was something going on I couldn't quite sort out. Mrs Gillick was behaving in a very youthful fashion and there was some impression I was forming, of which I couldn't quite get a grip. So I spoke instead with the doctor who had been on the platform supporting Mrs Gillick's point of view. His name is Dr Adrian Rogers and his moral position is to the right of the political spectrum. I said: 'Actually what is happening here is not so much an argument over children, because we obviously want the best for them, but about what the best *is* and how it can be achieved.' Dr Rogers looked at me with a bemused expression, and walked away.

I had only one other encounter with Mrs Gillick and this time it was by post, some time after the TV programme. When I was asked to write a book about the moral debate surrounding sexuality in general and young people in particular, I wrote to Mrs Gillick asking to interview her, for there was much about her that I didn't know and understand. I wrote the following:

Dear Mrs Gillick, We met once at Thames Television on the Sarah Kennedy show for a discussion of teenagers and sexuality. I am writing another book on young people and morality (following on from *The Ostrich Position*) and would be very pleased if you would consent to be interviewed for it. It will be published by Thorsons. I shall be discussing what is generally called 'The Moral Majority' and will be writing about your own role as a leading exponent of the particular views you hold. I would therefore appreciate seeing you. I am obviously prepared to travel to your home to interview you or else if you are in London any time in the near future perhaps we could meet then. The deadline on the book is fairly tight so I would be grateful to hear from you as soon as possible. Yours sincerely...

A few days later I received a reply. It was on a postcard entitled 'Corn Husk Mask of the Iroquois'. The picture was of a raffia mask in the form of a strange, rather frightening face. There were holes for the eyes and a large, hard nose, which looked as if it were made from some kind of extra-large nut shell. The reply on the other side said:

> Dear Carol Lee, Thank you so much for your most interesting letter. Funnily enough I too am writing a book. It's called *The Immoral Minority* and it's all about people with incredibly thick skins and hard *NOSES*. Do you know of anybody who might fit the bill, as you are reckoned by so many to be a leading exponent, etc., etc? Yours most sincerely...

I laughed, probably from relief, because suddenly the picture fitted together. One of the feelings I had about this card was that it had come from someone far younger than Mrs Gillick, and this gave me the key to her confusing behaviour with the young women that day at the television studio. I realized that it had struck me as strange because it was as if she were trying to make herself one of them. This could have been a deliberate 'image', because since she is delivering a Victorian message, Mrs Gillick may feel it would be unwise to appear too matriarchal. It may be that she decided her heavy-handed 'thou shalt not', 'forbidding' message would be unacceptable not only to young people, as it is for many reasons, but also to parents as well. So she may have decided to be modern and youthful in her approach. She follows in the footsteps of some highly successful eminent women if she feels image is vital. But my memory of Mrs Gillick is that she stood in the middle of those young women *trying to be like them* in a way in which I, who am younger than she, and work regularly with teenage girls, do not. This is probably why a number of them were nonplussed by her.

Many years ago I was asked to write an article on the late Enid Blyton. It was after the furore surrounding the discovery that her books were 'bad' for children and despite their popularity were being banned from some libraries. When I looked at them with an adult's eye (for like so many I was half-reared on them) what struck me most forcibly about them was that they seemed to contrive to block imagination, and imagination is one of the most precious, vital aspects of a growing child. The language of these books was unvaried and dull, and through this and other contrivances, such as the choice of situations and so on, the books ended up having a predictably deadening feeling. On reading through the hundreds of articles written about Enid Blyton I found, for me at least, the reason why. It was contained in the words of a psychologist who had interviewed Enid Blyton's daughter and had met Blyton a number of times. He said in essence this: that Enid Blyton was a petulant, difficult woman and that she behaved quite childishly on occasions. There were important things in her own childhood that were obviously unresolved so that in some ways she was still a child herself and that she viewed other children as competitors for affection and attention. She therefore subconsciously sought to retard them, to keep them back, and that is why she contrived to block imagination.

I subsequently found myself meeting the occasional person who suffered from what I came to call 'The Enid Blyton Syndrome' and knowing this helped to explain puzzling things about them. I noticed the 'Enid Blyton Syndrome' in a particular youth worker who, although middle-class, over-identified in a dangerous and damaging way with his perception of working-class teenagers. He 'talked working-class, like', and was over-accepting of the aggression and indeed brutality of certain of the boys — and girls. He was like a parody of the kind of youth worker who has got it wrong, the person who, in an attempt to make contact with today's disaffected youth, drops his adult values and behaviour and becomes *like a teenager*, or at least his perception of one. He presumably works on the premise that since adults have let kids down, one should behave as little like an adult as possible in order not to be rejected by the kids. What he doesn't appreciate is that adults have let their children down by not being adult and responsible enough. He has confused adult and responsible with being dogmatic and authoritarian. He also doesn't know that while teenagers want you to understand them they do not want you to be *like* them. They have quite enough difficulty being like themselves, *finding* themselves, without having the rest of us causing waves as well. Some teenagers seem to want us to identify and make comments like: 'She's just like one of us. She understands us, she does,' but they certainly don't want this as a way of life. Teenagers soon become bored with, and disparaging of, adults who imitate them. I suppose there are two broad types of people who do this: the ones who think adults have been 'too heavy with kids' and that what the latter need is someone to become like one of them, and those who by wanting to make their message sound less severe 'join' young people with it, rather than deliver it from on high. Both these kinds of people have mistaken imitation or identification for empathy, which is what we all want and need, whatever our ages, and both also have a subconscious need to meddle because of unresolved problems of their own. The youth worker I mentioned spent many years basically being bad for teenagers until he got 'burnt out' and retired to run his own business. After he'd done this he said:

> Do you know all that time with the kids was wasted. I wanted them to be like me when I was a teenager. And what was I doing but wasting my time? I told them school was a heap of shit, encouraged them to keep away from it. Yet if you ask me now what I would do if I had my time back again the answer would be 'study', jobs or no jobs. I'm not saying schools do a good job of the learning process, because they don't, but at least they give you a start. I'm really appalled that I've encouraged hundreds of kids to follow in my footsteps. Me, Mr Bigmouth. Yeah, I'd go back and tell 'em I was wrong. I'd tell every one of them. But I wouldn't know where to find most of them. Go on, print it. Tell the world Bigmouth was wrong. They'll know who he is, and maybe it'll stop other Bigmouths doing the same.

One way of looking at this man's 'confession' is to say that because he wasted his own teenage years he has made sure subconsciously that hundreds of others wasted theirs. He wouldn't do this now because he has moved on to being an adult at last, partly by reclaiming his lost inheritance of wanting to learn, partly perhaps through first-time fatherhood, for certainly he is the kind of parent who will make sure that his young daughter has the affection, books, play and exercise that she needs. But while he was a youth worker he was still an *unresolved teenager* himself which meant that he didn't, in fact, want any of the real teenagers to overtake him. After all, if some of them did, he might begin to feel uncomfortably as if there was something wrong — with himself.

Perhaps it is people with unresolved conflicts from their own teenage years who are the ones most drawn to intruding into teenage lives. It would appear that many people find meddling in the business of young people an incredibly 'easy' thing to do although I don't of course include teachers in this, or others who go through years of study and commitment. In a paper given at a meeting of doctors in March 1983, barrister Madeleine Colvin tried to make some legal sense out of the quagmire that Mrs Gillick. had led us into concerning parental rights over their children. While my own concern is with the moral rights the two are often closely related, and the following is an extract of Ms Colvin's collected data on the subject:

The practice of looking for parental consent is not and never has been based on any legal requirement: it has grown from the Victorian belief that children are the possessions and property of their parents and consequently had little or no capacity for self-determination. This in a sense was enhanced by the laws at the beginning of this century which punished parents for neglecting their children, for example by failing to seek necessary medical treatment. The second working assumption — although less frequently required to be practised — is that young people, where they are of such maturity, may be capable of consenting to their own medical treatment. Necessarily, this has been more relevant in those areas where the medical treatment impinges on a personal and private aspect of a young person's life. However, it is just as relevant, say to a 15-year-old who wishes to have cosmetic surgery for example... Fundamental to the issues surrounding the Gillick case is that of parental 'rights', 'responsibilities' and 'duties' and I will start first in assessing what these mean in legal terms. Perhaps rather surprisingly, although these terms are used in certain areas of the law, particularly as regards custody of children, they are nowhere precisely defined. Mrs Gillick is alleging that parents have (what appears to be in her terms an inviolable right) to supervise the physical and moral welfare of their children. It is true to say that the law does provide a tentative assumption that children, so long as they are minors (i.e. under 18) are technically in the custody, care and control of their parents. However, it is clear by making analogies with other areas of law, that such an assumption cannot operate to deny young people autonomy of judgement and to act independently of their parents in certain circumstances. The examples I am going to give may not at first sight appear relevant to the issues under discussion today but, in fact, they are relevant in showing that the law is quite capable of granting young people the right to act independently over major issues affecting their lives. For example, in criminal law, children aged 10 and over are, in the main, responsible for their own criminal acts and, perhaps as importantly, are entitled to arrange their own defence in the way they wish: i.e. in order to instruct a solicitor they do not need any adult intermediary such as a parent... This granting of independent control to a child or young person in situations where it might be assumed that parents would be in control has been done on the basis of a child's or young person's maturity or understanding... The courts have in other areas, such as custody decisions, given some formal acknowledgement to the reality that 'parents' rights' inevitably lessen with the increasing maturity of a child. The right of control exists only in so far as the child or young person does not have the right to control and as a young person gradually acquires his or her own capacity for choice, so parental rights diminish.

The point here is to do with the growing child's ability to use his or her own judgement, which is what good parenting is supposed to bring about. The obvious educational point is that judgement does not develop at the snap of the fingers or the wave of a wand, so it cannot be argued that it should be left until late in a child's development. The problem with the Gillick campaign is that it sought in a forbidding way to take judgement away from doctors, from teachers, from counsellors and indeed from young people themselves and give the right to it, at least regarding under-16s, only to parents. It upholds a system of ownership and of partition for it gives exclusive right over a certain *section* of the lives of under 16s to parents and not to other concerned adults. It supports an authoritarian system which views children as not having the right to judgement and parents as owning the moral and physical welfare of their offspring. It was most noticeable that, at a time when the figures on child sexual abuse were far higher than the figures for pregnancies among under 16s, and the NSPCC figures on child battering and neglect were running into tens of thousands, the Moral Right chose not only to concentrate on under-age sex but to try to bolster the rights of parents. Common sense, let alone compassion, should have dictated otherwise. Esther Rantzen's 'Childline' received 2,000 calls in its first 15 days of operation in November 1986, and the following month Dr Alan Gilmour of the NSPCC said that reports of sexual abuse of children had jumped by 126 per cent and that there was a 68 per cent increase in reports of children seriously or fatally injured in 1985 compared with 1984. He added: 'Our most recent estimates are that three to four children are dying every week following child abuse and neglect and there is now considerable public and professional alertness to the possibility of children being abused in an extreme way.'

The Victorian notion that children are to be instilled with our own values is not only dangerous to today's child, it is also a travesty of decency and of all religious values. If we propose that human life really is only a process of parents forcefully and forcibly implanting their own values into their children, then we really ought to stop pretending to be human beings and accept instead the status of clones. Certainly there should then be no pretence to religious feeling or motive, because religious feeling is based on the notion that there is an individual soul and that each individual is capable not only of working out what is right and wrong, but of acting on this. There is no point in saving an individual soul if the soul is not individual, and learning to be a moral, discerning person does not begin at 16.

The problem with taking on other people's moral development for them is not only that you dissuade them from knowledge and development which is rightfully theirs, but that you also run the risk of retarding your own. Perhaps this marks the difference between someone who is a do-gooder and someone who is a genuine reformer. The do-gooder considers it his or her duty to do good for and by others and therefore sets the clock of genuine progress back by the joylessness of this action. By genuine progress I mean that which contributes to our understanding of, and abilities to be more fully responsive to, our individual capacities as human and as social beings. The genuine reformer will instigate the abolition of the slave trade; the do-gooder will tell Muslims that the only way to God is through Christ. The reformer will lobby for a National Health Service; the do-gooder will minister corporal punishment to children saying it is good for them. I do not view Mrs Gillick as a reformer.

CHAPTER THREE

Whose baby is it?

The interviews I did during the time Mrs Gillick 'reigned' produced stories of moral dilemmas far more complex than the over-simplified headlines in certain of the tabloid press could capture. The underlying stories of many of them defied headlining and all that this quick-reference way of instant communication means. One such story came from a woman who works at a family planning clinic. She nodded towards a young girl as we walked through the waiting room and asked, after she'd closed the door, 'If no-one else has managed to educate her in 15 years how are we supposed to do it in a few hours? She wants a termination. You ask me about the moral issues of young women and termination. Well they're far more blurred than Mrs Gillick and the people who support her seem to realize.' The woman, who is in her late forties, explained that the girl had come to the clinic and had been verbally abusive. Sometimes this is a 'front' which young women put on when they are very frightened, and if it *was* that, this girl kept it up. The legal position had been explained to her and she had said contemptuously: 'Fought you was 'ere to 'elp people, not turn 'em away'. A doctor talked with the girl for a long time and she kept on saying: 'I want to get rid of it, right?' and was not interested in information which didn't support that request. As it happened, the girl's 16th birthday was a few weeks away and she came back to the clinic a few days following it, by now *demanding* an abortion and saying it was her right to have one. The girl *did* get a termination, and came back six months later pregnant again. This time the clinic insisted she go elsewhere for counselling and she was again verbally abusive.

The problems with which this girl presented the clinic seemed impossible to solve. The doctor who saw her told the story in some depth:

She was the kind of girl you feel like reading the riot act to and in part I did. It could be argued that she was not responsible enough to have a termination, but then she was certainly not responsible enough to be a mother. This is a terrible dilemma. I saw her twice, on both occasions for a long time, and in a way I was not surprised she came back, again pregnant. She didn't want to know about contraception and just said she was never going to 'do it' (have sex) again.

I thought quite a bit about her because she's one of the most taxing patients I've ever had to deal with. She presented me, and society if you like, with the impossible. I went up more moral dead ends over that girl than I've ever done before or since. For a start my attempts, and indeed my need, both personally and professionally, to help her she rejected. She made it impossible for me to get through to her in any way. She therefore dehumanized our meetings, when doctors like myself have spent a long time trying to humanize the whole medical process. So I was dealing with a set of circumstances rather than an individual. She was ferociously careful to ensure that I knew no more about her as a person when she left than when she arrived. She gave me only enough information to make sure that it was legally possible to sign a consent form to a termination and she only gave this when I said I would withhold consent without it.

What she particularly avoided giving me were any feelings. So on one level this girl should not have been recommended for termination because while she had *been* counselled I cannot say that she *received* counselling. She also brought out the punitive side in me because at one stage I wanted to exact the punishment on her refusing her what she so insultingly demanded. But where would that have led to? This girl, in her present condition, was totally unfit for motherhood, and would I wish to force this on her when it would result in a macabre punishment both of herself and of the unwanted child she would produce? The other problem is that this girl had already been punished enough. And I don't make that comment as someone who is soft on these girls because I'm not. It took me quite a while of being bothered by her to realize that you don't get to be that foul and unlovely without a great deal of hindrance and neglect. At one stage I felt like shaking her. She really tried my professionalism to its limits.

Then something else occurred to me about her, and while this might sound absurd, I think it's true. One of the ways she got under our skins was by arousing in us a kind of envy. She demanded things in a way lots of us would like to demand ourselves but are too well brought up or considerate to do so. She was thoroughly unpleasant to all the staff here, and because we're in a 'helping profession' she got away with it. I'm sure lots of the other waiting patients were envious of what she seemingly got away with. I've often wanted to be rude to someone but have stopped short because of my professional position or because of my sense of responsibility. And while the rest of us have the difficult task of behaving ourselves and getting little attention for doing so this girl steams in, does what she likes, and still gets seen. Of course her *actual* position shouldn't arouse our envy, but her drastic way of dealing with the system needles the kind of person who has quietly sat waiting half an hour for her appointment.

When you think it through of course it is dreadful that this girl must get brief satisfaction in this way. But only if we give it to her. By the time she came in for the second termination I had decided not to 'engage' with any of her bolshiness. So instead of being curt and angry with her when she rejected my genuine attempts to help her I quietly told her what her options were. When in the end she shouted at me: 'If I hurt the baby it will be your fault', I replied: 'No, yours. This is your pregnancy, not mine. It was you who refused contraception. If you want other people to help you you'd better start helping yourself.'

She calmed down a lot after that. I explained that I wasn't prepared to put her in for a second termination unless she had some counselling, and she seemed to reluctantly accept this. However she still didn't want to talk about the circumstances of how she became pregnant. It occurred to me that quite possibly the kind of sex this girl had been involved in is as tragic and distasteful to her as it is to the kind of people who get up and shout and scream about teenage girls getting pregnant. She was probably looking for affection, was *used* instead and then left literally carrying the baby while whoever had got her pregnant carried on his life as normal. I have no idea whether or not this girl got a second termination. I referred her for counselling and that was the last I saw of her. As I say, the moral dilemmas she presented us with are considerable. For instance, sex within marriage doesn't necessarily constitute a loving relationship. It was probably the case that this girl's parents were married, and what kind of job had they made of bringing up a child? The fact is that the vast majority of people are free, one way or another, to have children, and, barring infertility, may go right ahead. This is what we're stuck with, and the alternative to it, people not being allowed to have children, is monstrous. While people can go ahead and bring up girls as unlovely as this one, one might say that the least we can do is prevent *her* from reproducing, from repeating this mistake. But that leaves us on highly worrying ethical ground. I don't pretend to know what to do.

When I rang round some major hospitals to ask if counselling was provided for women seeking terminations the initial answer was 'yes'. However, in the vast majority of cases it was a doctor who did the counselling, not a trained counsellor. So the word 'counselled' here is used loosely to mean a chat with the doctor rather than in-depth or ongoing discussion and support. One doctor I spoke with even described the role of a trained counsellor in the case of abortions as potentially unnecessary because abortion was a social/political problem and not primarily a psychological/emotional one. When I pressed her on this she said: 'It's a practical issue. Women would stop feeling guilty about having terminations if society said that these were part of its function and service. The reason why women need counselling is because we still say 'abortion is wrong', even though we have facilities. Remove this and you'd remove the guilt.' This was the only doctor I met who expressed this kind of attitude, which I think is unequivocally wrong and denies so much that is morally important. When I spoke with a counsellor at one of the Brook Advisory Centres, where specialist counselling for women seeking termination is offered, she gave me many instances of decisions about terminations which were difficult to come to terms with. One was the result of an apparent case of incest. It concerned a girl who was 18 when she first went to Brook and who claimed she had been sexually abused by her father since she was eight. When she was 15 she became pregnant and told her mother about it. Her mother went berserk. The girl was removed into care where she had a termination. In the court case which followed the evidence produced by the prosecution was from the girl and her older sister, who also claimed the father had been abusing her. However it was the mother's evidence which won the day in court. She said that both her daughters were conniving and flirtatious and that they had drummed up the story between them. The case was lost.

When the younger sister went to Brook at the age of 18 she arrived with a social worker and said she was probably pregnant again, by her father. She visited him and they had continued to be lovers behind her mother's back. Both the social worker and the counsellor at Brook tended to believe this, the latter describing the girl, now legally a woman, was very 'biddable' and behaving like a fey 12-year-old. The young woman would not at first see the counsellor, but as the weeks went by and she kept on getting negative pregnancy tests she did. The picture from the counsellor's point of view was clear: the girl wanted to be pregnant by her father. She did not want to hear about the legal aspects or the medical risks.

The other person was a girl of 14 who went to Brook scared

that she was pregnant, as she indeed was. Her parent's consent was required for a termination and the girl's mother refused this. The girl's father had not lived at home for years and was not traceable. The girl was desperate not to go through with the pregnancy, but was made to do so. After the baby, a boy, was born certain things became obvious and the girl's mother 'came clean'. What the daughter didn't, and probably still doesn't know is that her own mother had had an abortion at the age of 19 and had always felt badly about it. She had yearned for the missing child, but her husband had left her soon after her daughter was born, so she only had the one child. When her daughter became pregnant therefore she decided that she could produce her lost child for her. Whenever the mother went with her daughter to the clinic *she* carried the baby. The teenager looked bewildered and lost. A social worker assigned to the case said that the girl was in quite a turmoil. In one way she was glad of her mother's help, but in another she resented her baby being taken away from her. The girl therefore was in a kind of limbo, neither fully the mother she had physically become, nor any more the young girl she still needed to be. When she handled the baby herself she did so as if he were a doll.

These three difficult situations show how impossible it sometimes is to find the right solution to such complex problems — even to find out at first what the real problems are. Do they then need our sympathy, or is it punishment we are calling for? That is substantially their moral difficulty. One of these girls might have been punished by *not* having a termination; another's punishment would be to be compelled to abort what she claims is her father's child; and the last girl's actual punishment was to be used without her knowledge to 'make good' a termination her mother had had.

It would seem reasonable to say that, because of these girls' youth, all their parents had in some substantial way failed them and that in one sense the parents are the 'culprits' here as well as the teenagers. The problem with taking this long a view is that it doesn't throw up neat solutions. It is not, for example, possible to punish these parents, even though the repercussions of their neglect and inadequacies will be visited on their children and grandchildren for generations.

If punishment is what we are looking for, then it's much easier to start with the teenagers themselves and say that if they hadn't had sexual intercourse then none of them would have been pregnant. The result of the parents' intercourse doesn't seem to concern us in the same way, perhaps because, in this case, at least two of the pairs were married. The girls however were unmarried and had made a wrong move that is easy to identify. At this stage the moral camp splits into two: those who say that, given these three girls' circumstances, in two of these cases abortion is certainly necessary; and those who say that (a) abortion is wrong and (b) in any case it is not the real issue because it wouldn't be necessary if these girls didn't have sexual intercourse. (The contention that the girl in the second case was an incest victim was not proved in court.)

The need to make sex outside marriage responsible for so much that is wrong in society, and for the breakdown of family life, is simplistic and spurious. The living arrangement called 'the family' has always presented people with problems. History is littered with copious references to and instances of brothers fighting brothers for thrones, fathers cutting out sons from wills (and daughters as a matter of course), husbands betraying wives and vice versa; all at terrible cost and with awful consequences. Family life has never been easy. What is easy is to try to find convenient scapegoats. If the crux of the matter is a family itself then we're going to have to look much further afield than teenage girls getting pregnant or sex itself as a reason for what we perceive as its present sorry state. One of the biggest blows delivered to family life in western Europe was the migration, in the eighteenth and nineteenth centuries, from country farms to cramped city dwellings — the Industrial Revolution, which ushered in the beginnings of the nuclear rather than the extended family.

There are modern parallels to this situation today in African townships. The problem is that to begin trying to undo the combined damages of industrialization and pollution is such a vast task. There are mistakes to do with land use, development, technology, education and the use of labour which would take decades of dedicated effort from millions of people even to begin to undo or repair. For one person it is an impossible task. One person *may* sit, however, with the help of a few friends, in front of a television set as Mrs Whitehouse does and start a national association which is widely quoted in the press. One person *may* start a national campaign concerning young people's sexuality as Mrs Gillick did. And as a result of Mrs Gillick's campaign young women (as it happens) were for a while more easily punished by unwanted pregnancy, and whether or not anyone wants to call it that, the way it is set up the word *is* punish. The problem is that the punishment creates more problems than it solves.

If a young girl is punished for having sexual intercourse by being refused a termination then the child she brings into the world as a result of her pregnancy is punished from the day he or she is born. The punishment of the girl who got pregnant is suffered not only by her but by someone who is innocent of her deed. The baby will end up either in care or being brought up by someone who is under strain or pressure and therefore more likely to neglect or damage the child.

But if it is *not* punishment we are calling for, then the picture looks different. If a young girl's unwanted pregnancy is viewed as a tragedy rather than a moral crime or a fall from grace, one works in entirely other ways to help her, and ourselves, for she draws heavily on our emotional and financial resources whether or not she continues with the pregnancy. For a start there would need to be the kind of sex education in schools where the subject of abortion was thoroughly looked at and discussed. Abortion would need to be looked at in its religious, psychological, emotional, social, medical and political aspects. The morality of abortion would need to be properly discussed, and the full facts of it understood, such as the difference between an early termination and a prostaglandin (which entails inducing premature labour). In the slipshod way that sex education has been ignored by adults or dealt with only partially it is all too easy, in the package presented as contraception, abortion and VD, for abortion hardly to be dealt with at all. The vast majority of young people I have worked with have been anti-abortion; by that they are against the idea of having or causing one themselves. A significant minority however have viewed abortion as an extended form of contraception or as a safety net, and this is obviously very worrying. But given that a full programme of sex education doesn't exist in most schools, much of the education has to come later — too late, in fact, in too many cases. Which is where counselling of people presenting themselves for terminations comes in.

The agencies that systematically provide abortion counselling are the Brook Advisory Centres and a few private charities like PAS (Pregnancy Advisory Service). And since Brook specializes in the care of younger people that is all to the good. However, because of lack of funding and therefore lack of staff and time to allocate to each patient, the time usually given to someone seeking abortion is only one hour prior to the operation and up to six hours afterwards. Most people do not take advantage of the latter. As a counsellor with Brook said: 'You can't *make* them come back, much as we'd like to see them.'

If abortion is seen as a tragedy and not a crime it is indeed tragic that girls cannot be given more than one hour in which to unravel the family, social and emotional circumstances which have brought them to needing an abortion. For there is a further tragedy which arises from inadequate education and counselling, and that is the small percentage of women who have more than two terminations. It is not rare for some young women to have three abortions and to keep on taking risks. One agency told me of a woman of only 27, a middle-class, professional woman, who presented herself for her seventh abortion, and another told me of a woman in her thirties, living on a housing estate, who had had nine.

The reasons for such tragic repetitions are numerous and complex. Too often, inadequate counselling does not allow for the fact that many women are in such a daze when they present themselves for a first abortion that they don't take in what is happening or what is being said, and go away and repeat the mistake. Too often also, many young women get a backlash of guilt and fear and try to test whether or not they can still *get* pregnant: try to test their fertility, which they suddenly think they may have lost. So in a sense they get pregnant again deliberately at a time when they're still in no better physical or emotional circumstances to have a child. A further termination only makes everything worse. Angela Neustatter, in her book on abortion, *Mixed Feelings* (Pluto Press, London, 1986), said that the women she talked with who had had more than two abortions tended to have extremely low self-esteem: 'It's something much more profound than being irresponsible, and with the counselling picture being so bleak it isn't going to improve.' Another common reason for young women needing more than one abortion is that, difficult though this may be to believe, some still don't understand contraception properly. After a BBC 2 television programme called 'The Trouble With Sex', on which I was a consultant, 2,000 phone calls were received from people mainly in their twenties and thirties asking for information. The programme was about sex education and went some way to illustrating from filming in the classroom what sex education actually is. A large number of adults rang after the programme simply wanting to know if there was anywhere they themselves could receive this kind of general education. One woman who phoned me through a friend two weeks after the programme was 24 years old. She said she was getting married in a year, was still a virgin, and wanted to know something about contraception. After half an hour on the phone she still didn't seem to be taking in what I was saying, and I eventually realized it was because I was assuming that because of her age she knew certain things, and she didn't. It became obvious for example that she thought the Pill affected male sperm, not the female body, even though she did, as it turned out, understand that it was the woman who took the Pill. She asked questions such as: 'But if you stop taking the Pill does the sperm get through again?' I thought by this time she was mistaking the Pill for a barrier method of contraception, but she wasn't. She thought that taking the Pill meant the sperm didn't get to the egg. She did understand that the Pill was swallowed, and not (as some other young women believe) inserted into the vagina, but thought that in some miraculous way it then had an effect upon the pelvic region to make the uterus rebuff sperm. And undoubtedly this fantasy was based on the notion that you only get pregnant if the sperm travel to meet the egg, so that the way you avoid getting pregnant is to stop the sperm from moving towards the egg. She hadn't understood that although the sperm *are* the major travellers, the egg travels as well, and *its* progress can *also* be retarded. I dread to think what a busy, over-stretched family planning clinic might have made of this young woman. But without a lot of help she and her husband may have been the kind of people asking for a termination a few months after marriage.

In discussing abortion with doctors, counsellors and young people, one of the most worrying attitudes was that of the woman doctor I mentioned earlier who thought that abortion was mainly a socio-political issue. A not dissimilar view was expressed by another woman involved in arranging National Health abortions, who said that multi-abortions were a social issue and that if women had proper housing and so on they wouldn't happen. I cannot accept abortion as simply a socio-political issue. I agree that abortion should be available, and yet I also agree that it is not just another operation, but the ending of an opportunity for a child to be born. It is one of the reasons why I call abortion a 'tragedy', and in defending it as a facility would also defend it as a major moral issue. Any attempts to de-moralize it I would resist. But if in making abortion freely available we have encouraged some, particularly teenagers growing up into adulthood, to view it nonchalantly, as just another National Health facility, then we have once more failed to take the time to allow its complexity to be discussed and eventually understood. It is this aspect, also, which of course gives ammunition to the people who have called themselves the 'pro-lifers' — a term which assumes that people who support abortion must be 'anti-lifers'. It gives rise again to the idea that the people on the Moral Right are 'right' and the people to the left of this (which is a very big space in the political and social spectrum) are nasty, immoral thugs. In thinking about terminations I would hope that there is no-one who would rather that they didn't take place. The long-term reduction of terminations can only be brought about by educating and helping women not to have unwanted pregnancies, particularly those who have many terminations, some of whom need concomitant psychiatric help. The irony of the pro-lifers' arguments is that they view termination as a personal sin rather than as a communal tragedy, and that their sense of responsibility for it comes too late in the chain. I would argue that the parents of the three teenagers mentioned in this chapter have their share of responsibility for their daughters' plight. But *their* shortcomings in bringing up three young women so inadequately cannot be 'taken hold of' in the way that you can 'take hold of' evidence of unmarried sex and say: 'That is wrong. Stop it.' A number of the young women I spoke with about abortion fitted Angela Neustatter's description of having very poor self-esteem. They didn't appear, on the whole, as reckless people trampling all over a system which had been too liberal with them, but rather as people who were paying a disastrously high price for trying to find out what it is to be a woman. I would even say that a number of them were testing their fertility almost as if it didn't belong to them, and certainly without being aware of it. I even suspect that a few took risks, again subconsciously, so that they could for a while be taken care of within a system which offers them the opportunity for a pregnancy test and a chat with a nurse or a doctor. They didn't know how to ask for more — perhaps because, in the main, we don't offer it to them.

The notion of punishing these girls is sometimes understandable because some of them can be exasperatingly rude, but it must surely be left there, as an understandable feeling, from which we must move on to the real work of skilful help. The idea that if a girl wants the pleasure of sexual intercourse without the responsibility you should then force her to pay the consequences, ends up down a blind alley with even more conundrums for the rest of us — not least of which is, where is the absent male in our reckoning? If she is forced to have a child, then we condemn the infant possibly to being brought up badly, and therefore suffering his or her fate at the hands of the punishment chain. If you say that the baby should be forcibly taken away from the young mother, which is what I have heard argued, then you bring an unwanted *and* motherless child into an over-populated society. The more you go down punishment alley, and think carefully about its possible consequences in practice rather than theory, the narrower it becomes.

Instead of this we could move towards trying to make sure that young people, boys as well as girls, are fully aware of all the implications of abortion, and that it is put in an historical context. I have been alarmed in classrooms so many times to meet 15-year-olds who have no historical perspective on what we accept in modern relationships. Children who have been brought up in an era where the Pill is commonly available often do not realize that it has only been so for less that three decades. It is not anywhere near enough to teach pupils today that abortion is available 'on the National Health', as if it were no more important than having a tooth out, for that *is* the way to attitudes which must give cause for concern. Unless contraception and abortion in particular are put into social perspective, how are young people to begin to understand their complexity? This is a further reason why proper sex education cannot be left to parents alone, for it is an historical subject and only attains its correct moral dimensions when viewed and taught as such. Sometimes, looking round a class of 14-year-olds, I have the impression that they have been what can only be described as 'jump-started' into the late 1980s, with no understanding of their beginnings and therefore little prospect of making sense out of the present, let alone the future. Most pupils are astonished to learn that the Pill is a post-war development. Somehow, without thinking about it, they had imagined it was always there. This distorts their view of relationships and reality by putting them into some kind of hideous time-warp. In an article on sex education in the *New Statesman*, 12 September 1986, Andrew Lumsden and Denis Campbell make the following point:

> Preparation for children (five to 16) for life as sexual beings among *other* sexual beings ('sex education') should be built around the largely ignored and downward-drifting history curriculum — which might help, and this is not a frivolous point, to *revive* history studies in schools. Half of all children today, it's estimated, learn no history after the age of 14... Teacher-training would have to be overhauled. The past century's massive body of work on evolving human ideas about its own sexuality is nowhere formally reflected in the education of educators. New classroom materials would be required from educational publishers. These would have to be most carefully prepared to avoid indoctrination, whether

53

religious or secular, so that classroom and 'pastoral' discussion of sexual issues would be better grounded in *facts* — supposed *sine qua non* of a good education.

Facts may not be *all* that the process of education is meant to elucidate, but in the moral and sexual education of young people there are far more facts to be reckoned with than most people realize.

CHAPTER FOUR

Trouble at the housing department

The idea that it is only girls who are involved in morality has many unfortunate historical precedents, and was given much current emphasis during the Gillick campaign. Although I'm sure Mrs Gillick must have occasionally mentioned boys she didn't do so often enough or with enough emphasis for this to show up. Presenting teenage pregnancy simply as a problem for girls, however, is insulting not only to girls, but to boys also. It reinforces the idea that girls need to be taken care of and boys will take care of themselves, and denies boys their rightful place in the process of moral education. It perpetuates the idea that they are morally inferior. This has angered some of the boys I've worked with, many of whom defy the stereotyped image of young men as being selfish and wayward. One of these boys said one day of Mrs Gillick: 'Does she think we've got no feelings or something? Of course the boy's as responsible as the girl, and if he's older than her he's *more* responsible. I don't know why people think boys don't care about these things. I tell you I wouldn't sleep at night if I got a girl pregnant.'

While sympathizing with this 16-year-old, I also felt it necessary to ask him to search his experience and memory for instances of men being less than responsible with women. I asked the whole group to give reasons why boys might or could care less than girls about pregnancy. But as well as the obvious work on boys' feelings and attitudes that you would expect this kind of enquiry to produce, something else transpired from this session for which I have to thank that same young man: for as well as anger, his original comment contains *jealousy*. Why should it be only *girls* that get a certain kind of attention? Why not boys too?

The result of this was that we spent a most rewarding time discussing how boys are jealous of girls. The accepted way of thinking is that the jealousy exists the other way round, that girls are jealous of boys' freedom, superior strength, better positions in the world and, post-Freud, of the penis itself. In fact, when allowed to, and when I have deliberately worked towards it, boys have expressed a great deal of envy of girls. They see girls as being able to communicate more easily with each other and as having easier access to a wider range of emotional expression. They also see them as having greater access to emotional warmth, to being spoiled (by still being cuddled at home) and to the kind of stability which the boys have been conditioned to think it is not masculine to want. This envy is a part of the reason boys take the initiative and start attacking the girls shortly after they leave the age when both sexes are cuddled more or less equally. Boys calling girls 'soppy' at the age of nine or ten is therefore often a way of trying to get back at the girls for what the boys subconsciously see themselves as lacking. By the time adolescence approaches it must seem to the pubescent boy as if many of the cards are stacked against him, which is why he develops such an aggressive approach to his own body and to his peers. While I'm seldom popular for saying it, it's the reason I continue to say that adolescence is often far more difficult for boys than for girls. The market place partly reflects this. Advertising for tampons, towels, bras and so on is commonplace in teenagers' magazines. Films are made to introduce girls to menstruation and into young womanhood. Altogether the sexual development of the young woman and its concomitant need for certain commodities is given a higher profile in advertising than the sexual development of young men. So the world outside already tells the 12-year-old boy that his female counterpart is more important than he is. She is worth wooing for what she will need to buy.

On a personal level the picture is even grimmer, because boys are abandoned to their adolescence, both physically and emotionally. It's extremely helpful to talk about this in the classroom, and to present and discuss the similarities and the differences, physically and emotionally, between male and female adolescence. It is also important to discuss what makes the difference between a difficult and an easy adolescence, and what effect either of these might have in later life. In a difficult puberty for example a girl may be terribly shocked to begin suddenly, without any warning, menstrual bleeding. The development of breasts, body hair, and sometimes facial hair, can be excruciatingly humiliating. For one of the most alarming changes for a girl can be the *shape* of her body. Children tend to have 'boys' bodies until they are about nine or ten: that is to say, generally, a slim, straight-hipped shape. The boy retains this shape, but the girl's may change dramatically into what one girl described as 'a horrible bell shape'. The accumulation of breasts and flared hips is not to many girls' taste. It is, in physical form, the loss of childhood and of simplicity, and unless young girls have a positive image and experience of womanhood (through their mothers) they may resent for a long time this awkward, complicated apparatus which is their new body, and ill-treat it and themselves accordingly.

Boys ostensibly have an easier time than this partly because they at least retain their general body shape and because they don't have to experience and cope with periods. They do however have to cope with the emissions resulting from wet dreams — and these can be even more embarrassing than periods. This is partly because they're so rarely spoken about, and partly because they make the boy so vulnerable. A young man of 22 explained this feeling to me when he said, speaking of his early teens, 'I used to dread going somewhere else to stay, especially to my aunt's. I thought she was smashing and I really liked her, but I was petrified she would see something on my sheets when she came to wash them, or see where I'd tried to wipe it off. Beds are very vulnerable places. I stopped going to her. That's the effect it had on me. And that was a tragedy for me because she was a really warm lady.'

Boys' vulnerability through wet dreams, and through emission from masturbation until they've learned to have tissues handy and so on, is considerable. In sex education much is said about girls' vulnerability when periods begin, where of course sheets can also be stained, but there are important differences, not least of which arises from the role played by the mother. It is no doubt still the case that more mothers change beds and do the laundry than fathers. With wet dreams the boy is therefore vulnerable to a member of the opposite sex. The girl is vulnerable to a member of the same sex who has had, and is probably still having, periods herself, so that there is here the possibility of identification and bonding. There is also the possibility of chatting about periods through talking about various kinds of sanitary towels or tampons, and so making them *shared* rather than just personal or private knowledge.

Wet dreams could also be shared knowledge, but probably because they have no attendant commercial use such as the sale of sanitary towels, there are to my knowledge no films made specifically about them as there are about menstruation. If one *has* been made, I hope it includes lots of interviews with boys and young men about the feelings wet dreams themselves evoke, and about the embarrassment and possible ways of avoiding it. One obvious way would be for men to take an active role in fathering, so that they can help boys through wet dreams and early masturbation in the way that mothers help girls with periods. Equally of course, mothers ought to help girls more with the topic of masturbation, which is knowledge that most girls are certainly deprived of. Men do find it easier to discuss masturbation, although I doubt that many men will find this easy to do with their sons.

I discussed this problem in an article about boys and sexuality for the magazine *Woman*: I discussed this problem

> Girls have the association with their mothers and with other girls over their periods and talks about make-up and clothes. They still have hugs from their mums and dads and are related to more openly and easily than are boys. They find, as women tend to, some kind of nurturing circumstances for themselves. But boys generally don't. They have entered through no wish or fault of their own a no-man's land of irrefutable physical changes which we don't seem to be able to cope with — which is why they can't. Thus, wet dreams, embarrassing erections and sudden mood changes — none of which are asked for — happen to them, and for the most part we pretend they don't exist. A letter I received from a man after I'd written about the plight of adolescent boys said: 'The needs of young boys are so urgent and so misunderstood. Almost overnight they have to contend with urgent, instant and burning desires unknown to them only a short time before. It must be nigh impossible for a woman, however enlightened, to understand how boys feel.' I agree with this, and I think that we tend to accommodate female adolescence better than male. The changes in boys leave us nonplussed — and them wanting. But what they're wanting is someone who has experienced what they're going through and who can help them — and how many fathers are capable of this help? Their need is for an emotionally mature father whose idea of masculinity is other than the traditional notion of the bread-winning man who leaves women to take care of the physical, emotional and moral needs of children. Boys need a father other than the kind whose idea of being a role model is to let his adolescent son know what a lad he was in his younger days and how 'these women' (meaning mother and sisters) are all very well (nudge, nudge, wink, wink) but there's a way of getting round them. Boys need fathers who will be to them what mothers generally are to teenage girls, able to identify with their often difficult and bewildering development as emotional and sexual beings.

It would be wrong, of course, to give the impression that everything is now fine for girls and that it's only the boys' needs we have to sort out, because girls get far too little help as well. But the substance of the argument is that men do find it more difficult to talk with their sons about 'private matters' than women do with their daughters. Partly this must be an aspect of the continuation of male competitiveness, the old stud-in-the-pack idea of the older man fearing the challenge from the younger to his established territory and virility. Partly also the problem is that men are relatively new to taking on an active role in fathering, and also seem to be more reluctant to be generous with their own vulnerability: thus their continuing alarm in tackling emotions like fear and anxiety. And oddly enough another aspect of the problem is our inability to discuss the penis. All sexual parts are difficult to bring into discussion under their proper names, probably because we're so unused to hearing them said. The word 'vagina' is no more alarming than any other word, but all the heads in a bus queue will turn round if you say it too loudly. However there seems to be something about the word 'penis' which causes even more offence.

It seems strange when phallic objects are so prevalent that discussing a penis, its workings and attendant pleasures and problems, is so difficult. One of the problems in the classroom or anywhere else is that the penis is so *present*. This is probably why discussion of it is shied away from. If it results in an erection, what then, especially if the person talking about it is a mother or a woman teacher? I wonder if fear of this happening is one of the reasons why the teaching of changes during puberty has sometimes had so little human relevance. In an attempt to make the subject as disconnected as possible from the human body some biology teachers make it sound as if all this happens to another species. As a result, so many teenagers do not remember what they are taught. I have thought a great deal about the problem of teaching boys, my concern tempered by the knowledge of how much the work is needed, and by humour. As with one young man who said: 'I reckon you could say, Miss, that you're never alone with your friend.' Another boy was able to confide that it was terribly embarrassing when his mother tried to get him out of bed quickly in the mornings. She would call him from the landing and come up and bang on the door if she didn't hear the floorboards creak in his bedroom within a few minutes afterwards. I suggested he ask her to call him 10 minutes earlier so that he had time to get up more slowly and still not be late for school. 'She'd think I was barmy if I did that,' he said, explaining that he liked his bed and had always got up at the last minute. 'In that case', I replied, 'say you've got extra school work to do and you'll finish it off quickly in the morning.' 'Nah, she'd never believe that,' he said shaking his head mournfully. 'She'd really think I was up to something if I said that.' I don't know how he resolved the problem. The way we left it, he was going to ask for a digital watch with an alarm for his birthday, and manage as best he could until then.

Attitudes towards the penis itself and discussion about it are very strange and full of contradictions. When the Brook Advisory's education department in Birmingham wanted to produce a pamphlet on the use of the condom, advice from the Department of Health was that an illustration of an erect penis offended public decency. A non-erect one was okay. This advice must later have been revised, there have since been books for teenagers with pictures of the erect penis. It is the disease AIDS which has made it necessary for the word 'condom' to be used publicly a great deal. If this has the effect of making it more possible to talk about the penis not as a tool or a weapon but as part of male sexuality, then that will be all to the good.

There is a great deal of benefit to be gained from talking about male sexuality in the classroom, and the kind of worrying, aggressive attitudes which are presented wouldn't be so prevalent if boys had more help at home. For far too many boys, becoming adolescent means banishment from physical and emotional warmth. A teenage boy is almost literally outcast, because some mothers don't *know* how best to deal with him, some are just too embarrassed to think about the beginnings of male sexuality, most fathers still aren't around, and many who are haven't the skills to cope. A further key here seems to be that adults cannot cope with male adolescence because it is seen as the onset of male sexuality, *which is viewed as potentially threatening*. So one is not dealing with the male equivalent of an adolescent girl, but with rampant male sexuality itself. I use the word 'rampant' because it properly describes the condition many boys find themselves in. It is a condition of fierce contradiction, dictated partly by the penis itself and mainly by people's attitudes to it. The attitude seems to be that the penis is dangerous. It is dangerous to other men because, if you'll excuse the expression, it is a flagship of real competition, and because not enough men have yet managed to make it other than that. It is dangerous to women because if a woman however inadvertently arouses it she could be accused of being provocative and might therefore land herself in trouble. Most parents therefore give up and hope the boy muddles through on his own the way most men have to.

One 17-year-old looking back on the years of puberty said, 'You've just explained something to me that's been a mystery for years. I couldn't understand why my mam went funny. It was as if she couldn't look me in the eye any more. It went on for ages. It's only lately it's got okay again.' Had this bothered him? 'I don't know how much it bothered me. Things were so bad and so much was going on inside my head I wasn't noticing all that much. My mam giving me the freeze treatment seemed about par for the course, the way puberty felt to me. It's a wonder *any* of us come out normal.'

Most girls will talk with mother, sister, next-door-neighbour or older girl about things like periods, worrying about their breasts being too big or too small, and not liking the shape of their noses, hips, legs and so on. Most boys do not talk to father, brother, man-next-door or older boy about anxieties over penis size or functions, or fears (which are prevalent) that masturbation will in some way damage them. What they do instead is mainly fool around among their own age group, another factor which retards emotional development at this age. A girls' periods mean she may now become a mother, a possible nurturer. It's as if we view a boy's erections as making him not a possible father but a possible aggressor. So the boy has now become potentially dangerous. Far too many boys go out and fulfil this prophesy. This makes concentrating sex education on girls, to the detriment of boys, not only absurd but perilous. If we are asking young girls not to get pregnant we must also ask boys to co-operate. If we say that asking for such co-operation is a waste of time then we are saying that they are incapable of considerate or moral behaviour. This is not only insulting to teenage boys but also serves to continue to make boys and men outcasts from those very codes of morality we would like to see practised. This is why the current trend in some schools towards teaching girls self-defence needs broadening to include the boys in an overall programme of sexual and moral awareness. In a mixed school, if girls learn self-defence then boys should learn *why* the girls *need* to learn it, and what might be gained, or lost, from their doing so. It is after all ludicrously short-sighted to try to 'arm' the potential victim without also trying to *disarm* the potential attacker. It breeds between young men and women further jealousy, resentment and antagonism. It is sadly still true that there are human time bombs, potential rapists and muggers in our schools, so isn't it logical to begin the work of defusing them while there is still a framework — the school — in which to do so?

Working with girls without working equally with boys, and without also bringing them both to work together, is extremely divisive and serves to put the double burden of morality on to women: that of being responsible not only for ourselves but for what others may do to us. It leaves boys in a moral wilderness from which they are far more likely to attack, for if you presume a teenage boy is beyond the pale he will do you the grave disservice of proving you correct. Allowing boys to dupe us with their some-times surly and aggressive postures into believing that they will muddle through on their own achieves the extraordinary feat of being sexist to both females and males at once. It gives women the added burden of being responsible for both parties and pre-sumes that men are not basically smart enough to handle their share of this work. It leaves the door open for some judge in the future to say a woman in a rape case 'Why did you not employ self-defence techniques when all the girls in your school had had lessons?' It also leaves the door open for a mother to protect her rapist son 'because he's not a bad boy really. *He didn't know what he was doing.*' Part of the work I do in a classroom is to *name* for boys what they are doing, and it seems that in many cases I am, for them, the first person to have done this. The names are words like jealousy, vulnerability, fear, need, aggression, and one of the subjects I talk about with them and time and time again is rape.

To talk about rape and the education of teenage schoolboys in the same breath sounds harsh, unpalatable and possibly damaging. It sounds as if I may be suggesting that I want the riot act read to a group of young people, many of whom are extremely vulnerable. But this is far from the truth. By discussing rape with boys I do not treat them as a pack of potential criminals, but as people who have been in the main denied the moral education due to them. It is also the case that this work with boys needs to begin in earnest if we want any improvement in our rape statistics. For by not accommodating male adolescence we are producing frightening, and actually quite logical, consequences. The lack of open, easy discussion means that boys are prey to their developing sexuality rather than being its host. It means that they are themselves easy meat for rumour, pornography and for gang warfare, for at least the latter gives them a collective sense of identity while their individual identity has been taken over by a nightmare called uninformed adolescence.

The progress of the penis from a relatively harmless water pistol into a fully-fledged 'weapon' with a mind of its own can be initially disconcerting to boys, but it needn't be a major disaster for any of us unless, by a conspiracy of silence, we make it so. Unfortunately we do. By allowing boys to feel that they *are* prey, and that they *are* outcasts, we make sure that some of them will eventually want to visit these misfortunes on someone else. By not introducing them to the 'female perspective' at an early age we make sure that there are certain things they really don't understand. One of the many personal understandings they don't have at the age of 14 or 15 is that sex with another person can be unwanted. They are so buffeted and conditioned by their own bodies and by their peers to the idea of sex as a 'going out and getting it' activity that the notion of sexual intercourse being genuinely unwanted is difficult for them to grasp. Here begins the idea that girls say 'no' because they are playing games, not because they want to say 'no'. This forms another link in the chain that leads boys to call girls names if girls have sex themselves. Many boys think girls are holding out on them from sheer bloody-mindedness and because it is easier for girls to say 'no' to sex. Girls are seen as having the upper hand; boys resent this and try and get back at them. The problem is that if these kinds of issues are not discussed right here, when the boys are young, many of these resentments will not be grown out of. And since research has clearly shown that rape is not about the need for sex but the need for power and the need to punish women, some 20-year-old rapists will be acting out this early resentment.

My experience in working with occasional all-male groups has shown that teenage boys find a discussion of this kind utterly compelling. You may walk into a classroom of 15-year-olds who are being rowdy and silly, and within 15 minutes the group has completely changed. The quality of their listening and of their engagement with you in the act of learning is quite extraordinary. They hang on to every word as if their lives depended on it — and their lives do. For in saving someone from unpleasantly formed attitudes about women you are offering him the chance of good rather than bad relationships, whether he be heterosexual or not. It is quite impossible, however, to work with boys of this age without using the word 'penis' many times, and without being completely comfortable in doing so. Having dealt with this you may then get on with other work with ease, but if you don't deal with it in the first place the rest of the work is hampered. They are so used to people not being able to do this, or to people doing it badly, that by the mere act of sitting down and talking with them easily and comfortably you have already brought about for them a minor miracle, and they are extremely grateful.

This is where having the time to separate groups by gender and then re-integrating them again is so important. Because the boys need so much attention, which they try to get by grabbing it, and being disruptive if they don't succeed, in mixed groups the girls can lose out, when they shouldn't have to. What is crucial is for girls and boys to be re-integrated after they have been involved in single-sex work so that both sexes can get more of what they need. The single-sex work very often lays the foundation for other work to continue at a much faster rate.

I've enjoyed working with boys, and perhaps one of the reasons is that the work is so immediately rewarding. So great is the need for this kind of work that any small help makes an immediate and tangible difference. So when I begin talking about unwanted erections, the myths about male masturbation (currently that it makes you not blind but impotent), the problems of competitiveness among boys, fears about penis size and function, the problem of feeling abandoned during adolescence, the pressures to be callous and brutal and so on, it is as if 20 suits of armour fall clanking to the floor to reveal likeable and concerned young people. If you then re-integrate the boys and girls you can begin important work on rape in particular and gender attitudes in general. While I am careful to point out that I don't presume people are heterosexual, I also state that often it is necessary to talk about attitudes to 'the opposite sex'.

One of the first things that becomes obvious from this kind of work is the earlier point I mentioned about the boys having tremendous difficulty in viewing any sex as unwanted. This initially brings out some flak from the girls who say, 'Yeah, they're always wanting it. They don't think about anything else', to which I reply: 'If you had penises which behaved strangely and parents who wouldn't discuss this with you perhaps you wouldn't be feeling so smug.' This raises protests from the girls that they're 'not smug, Miss,' and cries from the boys that the girls act 'very superior' and 'as if they're much better than us'. In one group this ended up with an eventual comment from one girl that she did in fact feel superior to the boys, as did most of the girls, because boys behaved so immaturely. By the time this was said a lot of good work had already happened so that it wasn't said with hostility or met with objections and resistance. What it did was to illustrate the original point we'd started out with, which was that boys got less help during adolescence than did girls and that this shows. It also enabled the boys to say how bitter and hurt they felt when they saw girls of 15 going out with boys of 17 instead of with them, boys of their own age. We were all now nearer understanding why. The girls told the boys that if they acted less stupidly girls *would* be prepared to spend more time with them, and the boys told the girls that if they acted in a more friendly and less stuck-up way the boys would not resent them so much. The boys were in fact jealous of the girls being more mature than they were. I was extremely regretful that having seen this group to this particular point I then had to leave them, for good. The subject of jealousy was therefore not taken any further.

Working in this way with another group we stayed with the subject of rape. One boy said: 'How do boys know what rape is like for a girl if girls don't talk to us about it?' A girl replied: 'If a girl even talks about sex in this school she's called a slag, so what do you expect?' From this polarized position the work began with me 'changing sides' depending on which side was being badly done by, and also acting as devil's advocate to illicit important points where they'd been overlooked. At one point a boy said: 'But a girl can expect to get raped if she's tipsy.' Oddly enough the girls didn't respond very volubly to this, so I did instead. 'So if a woman's merry after her birthday party she can expect to get raped', I said. He looked a little uncomfortable.

From this challenge a list arose, supplied by some of the girls as well as the boys. It said that a woman could expect to be raped if she was any of the following: bra-less; walking home late; wearing lots of make-up; wearing tight or revealing clothes and/or large ear-rings; looking very attractive; tipsy — and if she was drunk she could certainly expect to be raped. The list still took a while to unravel, but we did it helped by the fact that I was wearing large ear-rings, as I sometimes do. At the end we were left with a number of thoughts. The first was why should a woman 'expect' or deserve to be raped? What is there in our thinking, in our morality, which says that a woman might 'expect' this? Why do men really rape women? What is the likely effect on women's attitudes towards men if men are viewed as potential rapists? What could men do to help women and themselves? It was obvious that the boys *hadn't* understood the horrors of rape, and neither had some of the girls. The most surprising example of this was in a group of girls of about 15 who expressed the thought that far too much fuss was made about rape. After dissuading them from the idea that it was anything else than a very grave matter indeed, sometimes resulting in life-long psychological damage, I wondered afterwards why they'd held their attitudes. I could only think it was because since a number of them probably wanted sex, but were too scared of the consequences to go ahead, that they too had mistaken rape as being a sexual, rather than a demeaning, violent experience, In other words they had viewed it as a way of having sex without being responsible for it. I've discussed this kind of attitude many times now with teenage girls, for there is no doubt that some of them have an ambivalent attitude towards sex. They both want and don't want it. In a mixed group I tell the boys this in front of the girls, who are usually grave and silent at this point. I then switch sides again and say: 'Knowing all this I would argue that there is nevertheless no excuse for a boy to rape a girl' and (switching sides again) 'if there *are* girls who are deliberate teases, let's make no mistake about it, they are not only putting themselves in danger but causing bitterness and difficulty for other people as well.'

Introducing both sexes to the real reason why adult males rape women is also a very productive piece of information for them to work with. When I explain than men do this to degrade women, and to wreak revenge for their own inadequacies on people weaker than themselves, the boys are appalled. When rape is explained, not as a macho exercise, but as one which arises from terrible male inadequacy about sex and relationships, a pin dropping in the room would sound explosive in the deep thoughtful silence. When I further explain that the reason rape seems to be an increasing problem has a lot to do with men's reaction to feminism, in the form of punishing women for being independent sexual beings, it gives the boys a great deal to think about. One boy came back to me after we had been discussing rape the previous week and said: 'It was pretty heavy stuff, Miss, but it made sense and it made a lot of us think, it really did.'

The research which shows that boys grab a disproportionate amount of time during classes is borne out by my own experience in classrooms where the boys are aged around 14 to 16. Quite often by the time pupils have reached the sixth form this isn't happening any more. The ages when boys are grabbing attention are generally 11 to 16, the time when they are experiencing the most fierce sexual changes in themselves, and where they are jealous of girls who not only have changes which seem less fierce but who also have mothers, and each other, to confide in. The girls not only seem to have it easier, and grow up more comfortably, but they then look down on the boys to boot. It's no wonder, in these circumstances, that the boys decide to express their jealousy and outrage in disruptive ways. The question is, what are we going to do about it?

Altering bad habits at this age isn't anywhere near as difficult as trying to alter them ten years later. It would even be possible, if sexuality and relationships were really part of the school curriculum and began at the age of 11, for some very bad habits never indeed to form. One of these bad habits, which many young boys develop early on, is what I can only call a mechanical or technological attitude towards sex. They think sex is about 'doing things' rather than about feelings. Where the attitudes are really bad, and never challenged, it becomes too easy to substitute the word 'women' for the word 'things', and you have the progression from worrying to dangerous. It is not surprising, when you understand their jealousy and their continuing lack of care, that some boys think girls are for doing things to, and eventually for doing *in*. My value in the classroom is that boys meet a woman who does not treat them as if they belong to an untouchable caste and who is not pushed over by some of their initial antics. For the most part I've come to expect them. It doesn't surprise me any more if a seemingly unconnected arm suddenly rises from a sea of faces and, after risking severe cramp, one boy rises to join us from his position under the table. Neither does it surprise me when one of them keeps on lobbing in ridiculous comments like: 'I heard of a boy who suffocated from wearing a condom. Honestly, it got stuck and he died.' It is not surprising that young boys have this initially mechanical attitude. When you consider what the penis does, unbidden it seems, it is almost predictable that for a while it is viewed as a cross between the eighth wonder of the world and a hydraulic system it's better to be on the right side of. At this age it is both friend and foe, and it certainly behaves like and responds to being treated like a piece of equipment. Its antics, unless explained properly in sex education, are only comparable with what they learn about in the physics lab, and if men are 'penis-centred' then I'm not at all surprised. There isn't anyone around at this age to let boys know that their errant willies are not the centre of the universe.

It takes only an hour or so to do the kind of work which literally transforms boys' attitudes both now and for the future. Since they are so penis-preoccupied at this age you are, for a start, the first adult they've met who will not only talk about what most interests them but carry on talking about it! I start simply by saying that they imagine sex is about 'doing' rather than 'being' or 'feeling' precisely because a penis 'does things' in such an obvious way. I explain that this leads them into a mechanical attitude towards sex, which is a mistake. I further explain that women are not machines where if you push or pull certain parts of them the right things will happen. I also explain why a girl tends to begin her sexuality in the feeling world, and why boys do not. By the time we've got this far I'm usually deluged with questions, extremely sensible ones, and work continues from there. There was, for example, the boy who said: 'But sex *is* physical. How do you get away from that. If the bloke couldn't get it up there wouldn't be any sex.' 'Wrong', I say gently. 'Let's look at what sex actually is...' A useful way of introducing young boys to the fact that sex is not mainly physical is to ask each of them to clasp his own hands together. 'You are holding your own hands,' I say, 'and this is not sexually exciting. However, if you were holding hands with someone you were very attracted to we all know you would feel quite different. It's still your hand being held. And notice I use the words "you would *feel* quite different". The *physical* difference between holding hands with someone you're attracted to and holding hands with yourself is negligible. The difference is what you *feel* about that person. Isn't it?'

When enough time is *not* available, this kind of work can be counter-productive. I was involved in one session with the sixth form in a mixed-sex school which was, from my point of view, disastrous. I accepted the undertaking on the condition that a staff member be present to see what happened. I thought it better to accept just one session, which is not good for pupils, in the hope of persuading staff that the work was important. Never again. The damage done in classrooms is of many different kinds, and that day, by trying to move too fast, I took the girls along with me, but left the boys behind. I had for a start over-estimated the maturity of the entire group. They were a mixture of first- and second-year sixth and most of them were less emotionally knowledgeable than I had anticipated. We were talking about sexual language, which I felt was a specific enough topic to try to tackle in just one hour and ten minutes. We got on, very slowly, to talking about male and female attitudes to sexuality. And since I was beginning to notice how uncomfortable the boys were, I said that despite the girls' complaints about boys calling them names etc, it was boys who had a more difficult time during adolescence. That did it. The boys were so defensive by this time that this wasn't what they wanted to hear. 'That's a sexist remark,' said one of them, and with only five minutes to go before the end of the session there was very little to be done. To the casual observer this group would not have seemed particularly worrying, but I could feel the boys grouping to protect themselves as surely as if they'd built a high wall. While the girls wanted to continue talking, and I stayed with them for 20 minutes during break time to do this, the boys were furious that I had dared to try to expose their vulnerability. I, in turn, was angry with myself for taking the risk of doing what I had hoped would turn out to be an introductory lesson, but which turned out to be, disastrously for the boys, the only one.

In a previous discussion of sexual language with the fifth-form in this school we had ended up trying to find words for what the vagina did to, or with, the penis in an act of intercourse. Since we discovered that all the slang words we had for sexual intercourse were male 'doing' words like screw, grind, and so on, I asked them to try to imagine the vagina, not as passive but as active. I asked them for example to take the phrase 'give her one' and make it active on the vagina's part. That was turned round to 'receiving one'. So we worked out that the vagina received, took in, embraced, held, sucked and 'gave a home to' which we described as 'housed'. We found the word 'suck' a difficult one to use because, even though we all began as infants who sucked, they felt the word now had a degrading connotation. I understand why, and also expressed the hope that we would somehow find a way to reclaim important words, and not let our fear of our bodies make them distasteful. We weren't sure that we had learned anything from making the vagina active, although one girl suggested that by being aware of the vagina in this way it might improve our sexual attitudes and make boys behave differently. We left the discussion with this thought, and with a contribution from a boy who said: 'I take the point Miss, I really do, because you're talking about feelings and attitudes. But I'm going to fall about the next time my mum says she's going to the Housing Department.'

CHAPTER FIVE

I would like to walk barefoot through your hair

Having said it is often the case with a mixed-sex group that boys will try to dominate the proceedings, in one group I worked with it was the girls who grabbed the advantage by rather unusual means. This came about as a result of a simple exercise which I asked a group of 15-year-olds to do. It involves splitting the group into male and female and giving each a piece of paper and asking each group to write down what they like and don't like about the opposite sex. (I ask them to make sure the list of likes and dislikes is the same size otherwise you get mainly dislikes!)

Quite often you get a male/female split here, with the boys giving you a list of physical attributes and the girls mentioning things about personality and so on. This in itself is the first subject of discussion; the enquiries which follow on from it can lead to any number of places. One group of boys had on their list against the 'don't likes', 'They keep secrets' and the unravelling of this was a revelation in more ways than one. When asked what exactly this meant, the boys started talking about the way girls were not open when boys were around, that they laughed at the boys and then put their heads together and whispered things. But it went much further than that. Part of what they were saying was that girls had mysteries to do with their bodies which the boys didn't know about, and it turned out that these boys had never had anyone to talk with them about menstruation. So I decided to put this right, and the following week took in various kinds of towels and tampons to show them. Initially the girls weren't too pleased about this and we discovered that the girls in this group had been intuitively aware of the boys' ignorance and had deliberately played on it. They had played games of flaunting, of being haughty, and in fact of building up a mystique of there being girls' secrets that, do what they might, the boys could not find out about. All of this came our during our talks, conducted in a large circle. The words were their own, and my job was only to understand what they were saying, to realize the implications and to take them on a bit further. So, for example, when a girl said: 'Why *should* they know about periods? They don't happen to them,' I asked her if you only ever learned about things that happened to you. I also asked them all what the purpose of education was, and what they thought would be the end result in heterosexual or homosexual relationships if either sex was ignorant of many things about the other. It's unusual in my experience for girls to get the edge over boys in this way, for I'm far more used to it being the other way round, with boys grabbing the sexual advantage by calling girls names like tarts and sluts. So a simple phrase in a list, 'They keep secrets', had uncovered something extremely important, not only for these teenagers' present lives but for their future relationships.

I preface an exercise like this one by saying that it is a heterosexual exercise, and I like to follow it the next week with one which doesn't presume heterosexuality or homosexuality. This is where I also ask them to write things down on bits of paper, and if the first exercise has been a group concern, this is an individual one. I ask them to answer a dozen or so questions which go something like this: 'What do I like about being a boy?' 'What do I like about being a girl?' 'What do I not like about being a boy?' 'What do I not like about being a girl?' 'What do I like about girls' company that I don't like about boys'?' 'What do I like about boys' company that I don't like about girls'?' and so on. The list can be long or short, very simple or slightly more sophisticated. I've used it with adults and teenagers and I'm very grateful to the youth worker friend who first introduced me to it.

We often examine in the classroom the roles males and females act out and how they are for the most part so uncomfortably pinned on. I don't like clichés, so will seldom use words like 'sexism', which I'm afraid has become a jargon word for a lot of teenagers. What we discuss instead is how people may have a better understanding and clearer vision of each other. It is an attempt to re-introduce pupils to the knowledge that co-operation is theirs and is to be used. This feeling of co-operation among a group is important in all kinds of ways. It is sometimes best described by illustrating what happens when it's absent, not only among the pupils themselves but in other ways too. One group I worked with astonished me recently by *not* playing something I call 'The Word Game', which is an exercise in looking at sexual language by looking at the different, mainly slang words we use for sexual acts and parts of the body. When I say they didn't play,

I mean that they sat in uncomfortable silence when I explained that I wanted them to give me words they had heard or would use themselves instead of words like penis, vagina, sexual intercourse and so on. Since they were all 16 or 17 I was at a loss to understand what the problem was, although it gradually became clear. For a start we were sitting in a science lab with a high ceiling and a raised platform on which I had to stand to write on the blackboard. Many years ago I said I would never again work in a science lab, after a group I worked with had nearly started a riot in one. But given that there were two staff members present in this group, and that the pupils were of school-leaving age, a riot was unlikely. The problem *here* was inertia. As I waited for any response to my requests for words I became aware of how dreadfully noisy the classroom was. This part of the school backed on to a main road and the buses and heavy traffic trundling down it made a constant roar. At the same time I realized that ever since walking into this impersonal place my voice had been considerably raised to make myself heard. So I asked the group to forsake the safety of their leaning posts round various parts of the large fixed tables and got them all round near the front of the platform. There the work continued in a stumbling fashion. At the end of this session I turned to talk with the two staff members, and a girl popped her head back round the door. She said, hesitantly: 'You taught me last year, Miss. We were two different groups today. That's why we didn't say very much. People didn't know each other and we were embarrassed to talk in front of the others.' So that was the problem. It had not been *design* on the staff's part to mix up two separate groups and stick them in a large science lab backing on to a noisy road with a complete stranger and then expect them to talk about sexual attitudes, but it had certainly been default. In fact one of the two women teachers present said that she had complained many times about this room, which she found very hard to work in. The room was obviously not popular and therefore more easy to use as a spare room. School budgets and timetabling in themselves explain many things. Both staff saw the importance of having a far less intimidating place to work the following week, although the problem of having two groups together couldn't be resolved by this time.

I had asked for a staff member to be present because although I had worked in the school before, the new head of year had come back to me wanting just one double session. I explained that there was virtually nothing one could do in that time, but he wanted the sixth-formers to have something, so I agreed to come to the school as long as a teacher was present to continue the work if necessary, and to pick up anything from it that he or she felt was worrying for the group or which needed further working on. My request was also an attempt to persuade staff that dealing with the subject of sexuality, which includes sexual attitudes, sexual language, up-to-date information on AIDS and the effect an illness like this has had on both sexual attitudes and language, is a far more complex endeavour than they seem to think. But the combination of circumstances in this classroom had been a different lesson for us all.

What can be learned in a school depends on many things. School buildings and location matter a great deal, although I have also seen one excellent head teacher transform a foul-looking school, with the kind of prison-like environment that tends to punish the human spirit, into a place in which it was exciting to work. So while environments matter, so also do the qualities of organization and leadership and the calibre of individual staff members, although a lot of teachers won't thank me for saying this. They are tired of working long hours uphill when their work could be made so much easier if local authorities and central government viewed secondary schools as places of important learning rather than as short, sharp shock centres to equip pupils for the grimness of adult life. Where there are gifted, sensitive staff *and* pleasant surroundings, what is achievable in a school goes a long way towards encouraging the qualities of compassion and thoughtfulness. I'm thinking in particular of a school outside London where both the head of sixth and the head teacher have an empathy with their pupils which is lovely to see. When I raised an eyebrow one day at the comics in the Head's study he said: 'But they need them at this age. You see, the little 11-year-olds out there come straight from primary school. Some of them would run home to their mums and dads given half the chance. So if I see they're struggling a bit I bring them in here in the warm and give them one of these. It soon wipes the tears away, and they leave here smiling.' Rather different from visits to the headmaster in my own school days.

When I was working with the second year sixth at this school one term, they wanted to talk about emotions. As one girl had asked in a written question: 'Why don't teachers talk more about the emotional side of sex instead of just the bare facts. Could we talk about relationships because I have difficulty talking to someone that I like.' I wasn't sure whether she meant the second part specifically or generally. I certainly didn't know at this stage what the head of sixth's attitude to school relationships was. My feeling was that since these people were nearly adults we could probably work unreservedly; which we did. With a roughly equal number of young men and women present, making a group of about 16 people, it was exhilarating work. We began by exploring what avenues of communication were open to us and the impediments to them. They gave 'talking' and 'the way you dress' for the former and 'shyness', 'being afraid of making a fool of yourself', and 'not liking to be rejected', for the latter. When we went further into the worry about making a fool of yourself we discovered that this was quite normal. No-one wants to feel rejected.

Just knowing that this was common to all of us was a help in itself. We went round the group each speaking a sentence about rejection. I began by saying: 'I fear my writing being rejected because it makes me feel as if *all* my work is bad and that I'll never do good work again.' A girl said: 'I would be afraid to approach a boy I liked in case he didn't want to speak to me'. 'And?' I asked. 'Then I'd feel a fool,' she replied. 'Why?' I said. I suggested that all of us take the question further. Why do we feel fools? Some people came straight back to the word 'rejection' and I then asked: 'But what is so bad about rejection?' So eventually we got into the area of feelings. Rejection is bad because it makes you feel less secure; it can make you feel smaller. We also discovered that it has something to do with power. Part of the problem is that you feel the person who has rejected you then has the power to put you down. 'But do they?' I asked. 'Who really puts you down?' 'Yourself,' someone said. This we agreed on. If you are feeling good yourself then, within reason, other people don't have the power to bring you down. Then you can suffer small disappointments without being distressed. Once you start feeling bad it's as if you give other people power over you.

'What happens if you give someone a powerful gift?' I asked. The replies were that the person (a) takes it and (b) uses it, and thereby makes him or herself more powerful by doing so. We put 'power' to one side for a moment and worked our way on to self-expression. We had some voice demonstrations of how it is possible, for example, to say 'Good Afternoon' pleasantly, nervously, disdainfully or abruptly. We discovered that eyes, hands, body posture, mannerisms were all 'dead give-aways' of ourselves. So we went round this group again saying things to each other and working out what the other person *received* from what we were saying and how this was different from what we wanted to convey. We then did this with the specific intention in mind of 'asking the other person out'. This took a bit of organizing because we had to work out what exactly we were going to say. I suddenly remembered that at a certain stage when I was at school it was customary for boys to write you notes asking you out. Girls didn't have the same privilege, or risk. I asked if this still happened and was told that it did a bit. So we moved from working verbally to discussing perhaps writing a note or a postcard to someone. It was still so difficult to work out what to say. For example a girl's suggestion of 'I like your smile' was considered too personal and intimate and 'Will you come out with me because I'm really attracted to you' a bit too blunt. Eventually I asked each of them to write down on a piece of paper something they enjoyed or wanted to do with someone unnamed whom they liked. I stressed that the phrase was 'do *with*', not 'do *to*', and also stressed that I would ask them each to read out their contributions afterwards. So they had to be prepared and able to make public what they had written.

Once more I wrote with them, enjoying being part of a shared enterprise but also aware, however, of my need as a teacher to tread carefully the line between openness and professionalism. So I wrote: 'I would like to hold your head and stroke your face, for you look tired.' I didn't keep the pieces of paper they wrote on, so I can't remember them all. I do remember, however, as if they were written on my mind in indelible ink, two of the contributions. They were both from boys. One said: 'I would like to slip my hand under your blouse and touch your breasts.' The other said: 'I would like to walk barefoot through your hair.'

I could hear the clamorous voices as I stood at the day of educational judgement and was counted guilty of playing sexual pied piper to the nation's youth. I also heard the silence in front of me, and responded to it. Throughout the reading from all the bits of paper no-one had laughed or sniggered. There were a few empathetic smiles here and there, but there was no mockery or criticism. All of us understood the poetry of 'I would like to walk barefoot through your hair,' and I introduced them also to the thought of the barely hidden power in the message too. This led us back to our original talk about power and we learned something about good and bad power. I realized as I began saying something about this that one of the strongest emotions of all, that of 'love' or 'being in love' initially brought 'good power' into play. I also realized something else, probably because both the boys who had read out these two sentences had chosen *parts* of the body, as indeed had I. It suddenly occurred to me that what was so good about 'being in love' was that it encompassed *all* of you, which is why sometimes the world can literally look quite different when it happens. So I suggested that, in general, we concentrate too much on the bits and pieces of sex itself and on the so-called erogenous zones, to the detriment of understanding that *all* of the person is a mass of sensation and feelings given the right circumstances. I often say that I wouldn't still go into classrooms if what happened in them didn't give *me* a great deal. I had just learned another way of showing that it is feelings which determine a really good sexual relationship, and not technical know-how. My learning was only just beginning as far as this group was concerned. When I returned to school the following week the head of sixth was waiting to have a chat with me.

'Your session last week caused quite a stir,' he said, and as I looked uncomfortable he added: 'In a very positive way. The note about "wanting to slip my hand under your blouse" was pinned on the notice-board for a while which is how I got to see it.' I looked even more uncomfortable, and was then astonished to hear him say, with a smile: 'I think it was a message for someone, and if that's the case I think it can safely be said that it got through.' I asked what would have happened if a school governor or a visiting parent had seen it. He replied: 'We are thoroughly committed to working with pupils in a way which enhances relationships and their ability to form relationships. That's what life is about. The parents of this school support us in this. If they had any qualms they'd soon come and sort them out with us.' In talking about relationships in school he said: 'Its not unusual in our sixth form for you to see couples with their arms round each other or walking up and down stairs holding hands. That is what relationships are. You have them, and they're out in the open. I would never want a policy whereby if you have a girlfriend or a boyfriend you have to pretend in school that they don't exist. That only creates undercurrents which are disruptive because other pupils pick up on them. I think you must have a degree of openness.' I asked what would happen if pupils held hands in class. he replied: 'I wouldn't object as a matter of course. It would depend on whether it was a hand they should be doing something else with at the time. When I was teaching English a long time ago we were doing love poetry and there were a couple of pairs in the class. You could see them looking at each other and squeezing each other's hands. It seemed right. Sometimes you'll find that what concerns a class or an individual is more important than what you should be doing at that moment. In the end you've got to live with yourself and you don't necessarily need 'O' levels for that. Education has to address people's needs as they perceive them. Good education must address the concerns and the feelings of the people themselves rather than impose categories and views on them.'

The story of the English class reminded me of the time a friend told me of his experience teaching art to third-formers in Yorkshire. He said: 'There was a boy and a girl sitting about three desks apart and what was going on between them was bedlam. There was paint flying, water being sprayed, things being said. It was non-stop warfare. If it hadn't been a classroom and there weren't people in between getting wet it would have been comical. I've never seen anything like it. Then I learned from someone else that these two were 'in love' if you like, or very attracted to each other. So in the next art lesson I sat them together, and there was all the difference in the world. They were as good as gold. Not a peep out of them. I saw them squeeze hands under the desk occasionally and I let them carry on so long as they worked properly, which they did. It was a revelation to me: one minute things flying around and the next peace and quiet.'

Back in the sixth form that afternoon there were more surprises. They were subdued and I wasn't sure why. In fact, as it turned out, they wanted to discuss love-making in some way, but didn't know how to ask for this and were also rather shy and uncertain about *what* they wanted to discuss. Some people wanted to know about things like female orgasms and others wanted to stick to discussing emotions. Once more there was a male/female split with the boys asking for the technical knowledge and the girls for the emotional discussion. After pointing this out I asked them to call out the emotions they felt could be involved in an act of intercourse. I didn't specify what kind of act.

It wouldn't be most people's image of 'the modern teenager' to know that they gave 14 negative emotions and only two positive ones. They gave emotions like fear, anxiety, jealousy, insecurity, worry, pain, hurt, anger and further variations of these like 'worrying you might not do it properly'. The positive emotions given were excitement and love. When I went round the group asking them to take one of the feelings and speak a sentence describing how it related to an act of intercourse all but two pupils took a negative feeling. They offered sentences like: 'I would be afraid to make love in case the boy didn't want to know me any more,' or 'I would be worried in case the girl laughed at me because I didn't do it properly'.

This group of 17-year-olds very much needed to talk about love-making not just from a technical point of view, although this was important knowledge for them, but as something they were beginning to feel ready for, and also afraid of. This eventually brought us full circle back to the previous week's work because we found out that we are afraid, nervous and so on when, we think someone might laugh at us. If, however, we trusted that person, and could talk with him or her and felt that we were liked even if we did make mistakes, then it was different. So if the openness, the honesty, the friendships were right the love-making could become a shared *exploration* instead of a frightening and therefore often disappointing *test*.

Watching the group that afternoon it might have been difficult for many people to imagine there was work going on at all let alone extremely important work. The overall achievement in such work depends to a very great extent on the attention paid to educational detail. The first such detail for me is the importance of working in a circle, or something approaching this. Too many times I haven't bothered to ask people to shift all the tables and chairs because it is time-consuming and potentially disruptive and noisy. And every time I haven't done it I've regretted it. I find it almost essential to work in a circle because of what it states and achieves before you even begin. For a start it presumes that pupils learn from each other. When classrooms were designed so that desks were in rows other assumptions were being made. It was assumed from this arrangement that pupils were only there to learn from the teacher, whom they all faced, and not from each other. There is very little you can learn from the back of somebody's head, which is the lot of every pupil except the ones sitting in the front row. Putting pupils in rows presumably regimented them, but it actually also made discipline a problem. You can hide behind a desk, especially if you're near the back, and it is impossible for the teacher to see everyone. It is also not possible for most of the pupils to see who is doing what among them. In a circle everyone's face is visible to everyone else's and it is much more difficult to hide or to do anything without many people seeing. Of course working in a circle means that the teacher is part of the circle and does not have an elevated position on a platform by the blackboard. This is a more vulnerable way for a teacher to work, and it is also more demanding and enjoyable. You don't have props to hide behind and in a long term you find better aids to education.

One of the important aspects of learning in groups is that if it is done well pupils not only learn more than they would in a conventional classroom, but they also learn other important things too. I stress 'if it is done well' because working in this way is an art as well as a highly developed skill. Pupils may learn from it how to listen to each other, how to be co-operative and how to be compassionate. They learn to be tolerant, and the shy, quiet people who don't have desks to hide behind any more learn to become stronger. They learn to be challenging without being aggressive and how to be challenged without capsizing. They also learn that there is a common pool of knowledge between them which can be built on to their mutual benefit and that it does not need a teacher to be present for them to learn from each other. They eventually learn how not to give away more of themselves than they should and how to survive if they occasionally do. Not only is this kind of learning crucial in enabling teenagers to become mature, loveable and loving people, but it also encourages the learning we usually equate with the classroom, the *subject* learning, to take place more rapidly, and more easily. Because the subject learning takes place less rigidly and more personally it assumes more individual meaning and is therefore better remembered. However, it is the word 'easily' that many adults have problems with. Remembering our own school days it is a problem to put the words 'easy' and 'lessons' together, for the learning was painful — and it was meant to be. If it wasn't difficult what was the point in having tests and exams in it and giving awards and certificates to those who deserved them? There is a fear that in the kind of group work I am describing there is little discipline and that any unskilled person could just go in and chat. In other words, it is not *work*.

As an adult I have been tremendously interested in and rewarded by the subject of history. It also interested me at school, but I found it difficult. I continued to take it through 'A' levels, getting only just above pass marks the higher I went and the more I had to remember. It was a difficult decision as to whether I'd continue to take it at teacher training college, and I eventually took it as a subsidiary subject for a term. I was very anxious about doing so, for if the history lecturer taught in the same way as my last history master I would be sunk. I had found him impossible to learn from, and had done what little work I could by reading books.

I can't unfortunately remember the name of the woman who took me for history, because we were only together for a term, but I *do* remember what she did for me and am continuingly grateful to her. She had been on a dig at Knossos in Crete with

Sir Arthur Evans and she showed us slides of this while she chatted animatedly about ancient Greece, about modern Crete and about the controversy surrounding Sir Arthur's renovation of Knossos. I thought I had arrived in an educational paradise. I couldn't wait for lectures to begin and didn't want them to end. I can almost say that my difficulty with history was resolved immediately. Passing exams became unimportant compared with the excitement of my new ability to make history my own and to make my own sense and connections from it. So I had been introduced to a personal skill by a woman who showed me the beginnings of what it meant to have an enquiring mind.

Equating work with words like 'difficult' and 'unpleasant' is not of course entirely wrong, for work is, in part, both of these, as many activities can be. Anyone who has climbed a mountain to get a spectacular view or drunk a little too much at a party knows this. It is difficult to climb a mountain and unpleasant to have a hangover. What makes the difficult aspects worthwhile is the personal need, and the short or long-term achievements. In his excellent work on education, the philosopher A. N. Whitehead describes both teaching and learning as happenings in three stages: romance, precision and generalization. By this he means that in the first stage, romance, it is vital to capture the pupil's interest and imagination, for without this education will not begin. In the next stage it is vital that the educator has precise information to give as a result of the interest aroused. In the third stage pupils then learn how to form connections, how to link up what they know to other topics, subjects, thoughts and feelings, and how to form general principles out of particular pieces of knowledge. By neglecting the initial romance stage, and going straight on to precise facts given out in a dry, unpleasant way, a vital stage in learning is missed. That important, first step is too often over-looked. When they are toddlers, children learn about the world through an unending supply of curiosity. While the repeated question 'why?' at a certain stage in a young child's life can be irritating, before this phase begins a toddler's ability to become absorbed or fascinated by an object or a task is extremely appeal-ing. Good parents and teachers use this natural curiosity as much as possible, as well as its concomitant ability to find the simplest things absorbing. When children are fascinated by objects, or point at things, like cars or flowers, we tell them what they are and sometimes explain them. So we name them, and the child is involved in a piece of learning and begins to use the word 'car' or 'flower'. Barring illness or hindrance, all children do this, and it is a natural, almost effortless process. If learning in young children were incredibly difficult they would not be able to undertake it, and would therefore not develop. Learning at an early age happens at the child's own pace. We name things when they point at them, we help them to walk when they are ready for it, and they walk, talk, crawl at slightly different ages, according to the individual child.

If you interchange the words 'curiosity and 'romance' Whitehead's meaning becomes clear. Toddlers are in love with the world which is why they want to find out all about it. As in any romance, they have their set-backs, disappointments and periods of boredom. But essentially, unless they are dissuaded from it by neglect or abuse, they are engaged in a love affair with this wonderful new experience of being alive. This is the main reason they are so appealing and why they also make us sigh and say: 'It won't last long. They'll soon learn it's not all sunshine and roses.' The wonderful feeling, in other words, of innocence, of being in love with life, will soon be replaced by getting to know life 'better', getting to know that it is also a hard and difficult business. The romance will soon be over and life will be seen, not as exciting and a source of delight but as a difficult endeavour. Whitehead suggests that the love affair of learning is continuable, but that if we make it difficult by taking away the stage of romance or curiosity then we lose the desire and vital energy to engage in it. The puritan idea that unless something is difficult it is not worthy is not therefore the whole or even the main story. Learning does become more difficult as one gets older, which is all the more reason why interest and personal need are vital to the process. If we can make more and more exploration and learning possible, we bring about the possibility of greater awareness, intelligence, sensitivity and love of life — surely no bad thing.

Making the work of learning difficult without allowing it to be accessible through romance or curiosity is a perverse act which continues an elitist system in which a few people called experts are 'clever' or knowledgeable and the rest of us are not. When you put together this puritan notion of learning having to be difficult to be worth achieving with the subject of sexuality, some of the reasoning behind the resistance to sex education becomes clearer. Basically sexuality is not thought of as being a proper subject. The kind of group work I have described, which appears simply to be people sitting around just having a chat, is therefore thought of merely as having a pleasant time, not *working*, as though these were necessarily different. It would be worthwhile therefore to summarize at this point the overall aims of these group sessions:

To encourage people to be considerate and co-operative.

To encourage personal and social understanding and responsibility.

To help reduce incidence of rape and sex crimes.

To make sure the medical, moral and social implications of AIDS are discussed.

To explain all contraception as a joint concern.

To explain the workings of male and female reproductive systems.

To explore the physical, emotional, religious, moral and medical aspects of sexuality.

To give an historical basis to male and female roles, contraception, abortion and relationships generally.

Not to discriminate against disability, homosexuality or certain religions.

To deal with pupils' individual concerns as presented, and where necessary translate through role play and exercises into general meaning.

To answer problems sensitively and be aware of hidden or other meanings.

To make sure certain subjects are aired if not volunteered — incest, abortion, common myths, menopause, the dangers of pornography, sexually transmitted diseases, etc.

To make connections with other subjects such as mathematics, English, geography, history, biology and chemistry.

To increase pupils' ability to use their own judgement and think for themselves.

To use rich and varied language in all this to encourage pupils' literacy and powers of self-expression.

To encourage self-understanding, and through this the qualities of affection, loyalty, tenacity and the spirit of enquiry.

There are indeed ways of sitting down and having a chat with teenagers without these aims in mind. But if you are a teacher paid to educate then these are just some of the things you are there to do, and it is your job to do your best to achieve them. The searching for new and better ways to do this is part of what makes the work stimulating, and many of those ways come from listening to the pupils themselves. What it is possible to achieve in the classroom depends therefore not only on the pupil's ability to listen, but also on the teacher's.

CHAPTER SIX

What the jury didn't know

As I was working in this way with pupils in schools, the October 1986 Education Debate was drawing near. Shortly before the debate, I was asked to be on a Radio 4 programme called *You the Jury*. As I hadn't heard the programme before, the producer explained it to me. He said it was a courtroom format for discussing topical issues, with the 'prosecution' and the 'defence' each laying out their arguments in front of an invited audience. The prosecution presented a case and brought two witnesses to support it. The defence argued against this case, also with two witnesses in support, and the jury decided who had won. On the programme both speakers got the chance to give an opening talk of one minute and a summing up of three minutes. They also had the opportunity to cross-examine each other's witnesses. The prosecution's case, led by Peter Bruinvels, then Conservative MP for Leicester East, was to be 'Sex education corrupts the young' and I was to speak against this. At least that's what I was told. In the few days between being invited to defend this and actually going on air the motion was changed at least half a dozen times. At one stage it stood at: 'Sex education can corrupt and deprave' which I said I couldn't possibly argue against. Most things *can* be bad for you if taken, for example, in the wrong way or too often, and while sex education is a good thing, it *could* be bad if taught by the wrong person. A few hours before going on air the motion finally stood at 'Sex education tends to deprave and corrupt', and this is what I was to argue against.

Mr Bruinvels invited Valerie Riches and Barbara Robson to be his witnesses. I invited Anna Raeburn and Michael Pipes. Valerie Riches was introduced by Dick Taverne, the programme's chairman, as National and Honorary Secretary of Family and Youth Concern, and wife, mother and qualified social worker. Barbara Robson was introduced as secretary of the Campaign for the Improvement of London Teaching Standards and as having four daughters all being educated at inner London schools. Anna Raeburn was introduced as author, broadcaster and journalist and Michael Pipes as Headmaster of the City of Portsmouth Boys' School and Vice President of the National Association of Head Teachers. It was not said at the time how many children Anna and Michael had. In fact both are married, Anna with one child and Michael with three. Peter Bruinvels' interests were given as politics and religion. I was not asked what mine were.

Mr Bruinvels opened the debate with the following:

Sex education is fast becoming a mass of conflicting ideas and ideologies. Gone are the days of human biology where uncompromising lectures on human reproduction were acceptable. Instead we have some teachers promoting their own sexual preferences, prejudices and proclivities, giving talks on their own sexual morality in such a way as to encourage young children to accept the abnormal as normal. Controversial side issues such as homosexuality, sexual promiscuity and other deviant sex relationships are causing parents and some teachers great and natural concern. Irresponsible and unpoliced sex education lessons are certainly encouraging children to possibly experiment and put this new knowledge into practice, a knowledge which certainly will corrupt. Sex education must be balanced, responsible and given in such a way so as to encourage all children, who are after all very impressionable at such a young age, to lead decent and happy family lives.

My own opening contribution was the following:

I will argue that sex education is important to the physical, moral and emotional development of young people and that it is the absence of good sex education which makes depravity and corruption more possible, not the presence of it. Sex education in essence is about allowing a young person to knowledge of him or herself as a complete person. I would describe this knowledge as children's rightful inheritance, and their insurance against harm. The harm comes from the flourishing business of pornography, the titillation of 'Page Three' girls, and the millions a year made from advertising, video nasties, and in places like Soho. Capital is indeed made out of our sexual and emotional insecurities, griefs and inadequacies. I would also say that there is no present substitute for sex education in schools, since to our collective shame most of the harm done to children takes place not in the classroom but outside it in a complex and very demanding world.

Reading back over that many months after speaking it, it seems a reasonable opening — but what the prosecution presented as so-called evidence astounded me. What is certainly true is that if Jenny hadn't been living with Eric and Martin at the time, at any rate in Haringey and Ealing, I really don't know what Mr Bruinvels would have done. The book which described how a girl of five called Jenny lived with her father Martin and his boyfriend Eric, had been hitting the headlines in the weeks leading up to the Education Debate. Given what it did for the Moral Right it wouldn't have surprised me if they'd published it themselves. As it happens, *Jenny lives with Eric and Martin* was published by Gay Men's Press in December 1983, and it was most fortuitous for Mr Bruinvels that it came to the public's notice when it did. This, and Ealing's and Haringey's announcement that they wanted 'positive images' of homosexuality to combat a heterosexist bias in schools certainly set the pigeon among the cats. The pigeon in this case was sex education and all the people who had ever opposed it licked their paws and gathered for the kill.

When Mrs Riches was called to the microphone she said: 'With the epidemic of AIDS, cancer of the cervix, rise in teenage pregnancies, rise in promiscuity, it is important that children learn about sex within the context of a loving family.' She then went on to mention three sex education books which contained disagreeable and damaging material, one of which was Jane Cousins' *Make it Happy* (Virago, 1978). Of this book Mrs Riches said: 'It encourages children to believe they can masturbate with kitchen furniture. Communal masturbation, group sex, oral and anal intercourse is very popular, and incest and even sexual activity with animals short of actual coupling.' She went on to say that the book 'puts into children's minds concepts that normally wouldn't occur to an adolescent.' This is where the trouble began for me, because having read Jane Cousins' book many years before I couldn't remember it stating these things, but how was I to refute in a few minutes what Mrs Riches had just said? Even with the book in front of me it would have taken ages to wade through it and describe what it actually *had* said.

There were other problems with Mrs Riches' 'testimony' that were difficult to come to grips with in a few minutes of cross-examination. She throws in a 'rise in teenage pregnancies' along-side AIDS and cancer of the cervix — a return to the numbers game. Teenage pregnancies are not generally rising. It would indeed be correct to say that teenage pregnancies have risen since 1940. But, again, without figures in front of me, there was little

I could do about arguing this. As I tried to think my way round all these things I remembered that Jane Cousins' book did describe the *meanings* of such things as bestiality and incest, but that in itself is surely not wrong. In a dictionary there are words like 'terrorist', 'fascist', 'torture', 'depravity' and so on. I trust that no-one would suggest that dictionaries should be banned because they give the meanings of unpleasant acts or people. But perhaps the descriptions in *Make It Happy* were salacious ones, so after the programme I read the book again. I could find no mention whatsoever of masturbation with kitchen furniture, and Jane Cousins, when I spoke with her about this, said there was no mention of it in any edition of her book. I did find mention of communal masturbation which was the following:

> 'Masturbating is usually a very private thing, although some girls and boys sometimes get a kick out of doing it in a group. If that's how you enjoy it there's nothing wrong in sharing sex in this way. If, as most people do, you prefer wanking in private, the big fear can be that you'll be discovered by your parents or by someone whom you don't want to know. If you should be interrupted, and whoever it is that disturbs you looks horrified, try to figure out why they are horrified. It could well be that they disapprove altogether, in which case you'll have to find a more private place in future. Or it could be simply that *they're* upset that *you* might be upset to be discovered doing something you wanted to do in private.'

I also found a reference to group sex in the following line: 'There are couples who like to be alone and those who enjoy sex with a group of people.' Nothing further was said about this anywhere else in the book. Oral and anal intercourse were discussed in more than one context, although incest was mentioned only in one section lasting less than a page. In this it was described as 'not particularly uncommon' and as 'a serious crime'. There is one mention of bestiality, a five-line description, which on reflection I cannot endorse or condone. It states:

> Some people feel sexually attracted to animals. It's not against the law to kiss, masturbate, or be masturbated by an animal. But it is illegal for a woman or a man to have intercourse or buggery with an animal. It's totally impossible for a woman to get pregnant by having sex with an animal — or for an animal to get pregnant by having sex with a man.'

With the exception of this last item, there is nothing here which could be said to 'encourage' any of these activities. It is surely better that such difficult problems are discussed openly, for young people *are* curious about such things, whatever innocence people like Mrs Riches may imagine. Not infrequently I have been asked about bestiality or 'sex with animals' by teenagers. For some reason it is a question which recurs, and was doing so long before *Make It Happy* was first published. In answer to questions I have given factual information and also the moral opinion that I think it is unnecessary, degrading and perverted. There *are* criticisms to be made of *Make It Happy*, certainly, but Mrs Riches' interpretation of the book is not so much criticism, which she is entitled to, as misrepresentation. However, it was the subject of incest which I was particularly concerned about when I asked Mrs Riches in cross-examination about the plight of children involved in this practice. Since incest happens in the home what would be the position of children if sex education were left to parents? Mrs Riches replied: 'I am aware of the problem of incest and I would say it is largely due to the promotion of incest, not only in sex education, but in pornography.' So Mrs Riches was saying that sex education, along with pornography, is responsible for incest, which is an extraordinarily convoluted way of protecting the icon of parents as always good. As it happens, sex education of any other than a purely reproductive kind wasn't even tentatively begun in schools until the early 1970s. The parents of today's incest victims could not therefore claim to have learned 'how to commit incest' from sex education in school. Although they could of course have been subjected to pornography. But Mrs Riches' juxtaposition of words gives the added weight of the crime of incest to sex education, which wasn't around when the parents of today's 15-year-olds were themselves schoolchildren. When you couple this with Mrs Riches' suggestion that incest is 'put into children's minds' by books like *Make It Happy*, this brings about a dangerous allusion that it is the *child* who is the cause or the perpetrator of incest not the adult. It is almost as if she were saying that by having knowledge of the existence of incest, *children* are more likely to make it happen, when it is in fact the adults who are the perpetrators. For even if a child were to behave seductively it is still absolutely the parent's duty not to take advantage of this.

When I asked Mrs Riches again about incest she replied: 'You know, what you're doing is taking a problem in society and sort of manifesting it over the healthy majority of society. It's a very dangerous practice. Hard cases make very bad laws and policies indeed.' Ye gods! She had just been allowed to get away with condemning sex education by mentioning on air three books, one somewhat inaccurately, and now scolded me about hard cases. The Moral Right's refusal to come to terms with incest and child neglect because its case rests on the sanctity of the family is a betrayal of children's suffering. Incest and NSPCC reports are not about a few 'hard cases'.

Continuing my cross-examination of Mrs Riches I then asked if she felt that topics like 'incest', 'masturbation' and 'contraception' should not be part of sex education. She replied: 'I think if a child raises these questions in class that child needs very special individual help...' There was some adverse audience reaction to this and Mrs Riches then added 'as indeed most children do.' She continued: 'I think the problem is that there's such stress on the negative aspects of sexuality that we're not reaching out to youngster's idealism and giving them all the positive aspects of sex in the context of marriage and family life.' I asked if she did not consider masturbation an ordinary human activity and she replied: 'I'm not talking about what you regard as ordinary. I'm talking about people saying to young people that if they don't masturbate they won't have happy sexual lives later.'

It is odd and somewhat unnerving, to be accused of things one doesn't do. What Mrs Riches had just said was not compatible with any of the work I do or have done in classrooms, and was certainly not compatible with the amount of effort spent trying to discuss masturbation properly. Only a few days previously I had talked to a group of boys about masturbation, and explained that it was not compulsory, but neither was it shameful, and that it had its advantages and its dangers. I had taken a great deal of care to explain that masturbation was a normal activity, but also that it wasn't abnormal *not* to want to do it either. I had also explained that masturbating occasionally was fine, and that sometimes one needed to masturbate more often, but that the dangers of masturbating too often were that you could get into fixed habits and lose some of your ability to be fully receptive to a lover, and that it was also important not to develop what I called 'a fixed fantasy'. Understandably the boys had dozens of questions to ask as a result of this extremely mixed message, and in answering each one I had to think extremely carefully about my use of language and emphasis so that I didn't give a wrong impression. I was eventually saved by a good-humoured comment from one boy who, after I'd replied to a question with something about being in touch with *all* of yourself, riposted: 'He's never out of touch with himself, Miss.' There were loud guffaws of laughter. After smiling at the joke myself, I managed to regain some ground by saying: 'There are more ways of being in touch with yourself than you realize, and most of them are not physical.'

After Mrs Riches, Mrs Barbara Robson spoke. If I thought what had already been said was distorted, then what was to come made Mrs Riches' comments seem positively benign. I didn't in fact put all the pieces of Mrs Robson's 'evidence' into place until some weeks after *You the Jury* went on the air, and then only by a fortunate coincidence. Mrs Robson had the following to say about her campaign for the improvement of London teaching standards:

> We were overwhelmed with parents, teachers and even children approaching us with problems to do with sexual education in London schools and also the immoral aspects and the lack of spiritual care that was going on in London schools. The sort of thing my daughter has been doing in personal and social education is cutting out pictures of naked women and sticking on men's heads. She's also been told she can get contraceptives without telling me: she was 13 years old at the time. In another class a list of questions was written up on the board for girls to answer. The teacher actually went round the classroom asking individual girls the questions and one of them was: 'do you enjoy looking at photographs of naked men?' The girl who was asked that question was a Muslim girl. She very bravely refused to answer her teacher and said it was against her religion. She was also given a leaflet which not only told her that she could drink at five, buy a gun at 14 and that boys couldn't be convicted of rape till they were 14: she was also told that she could leave home and enter a brothel at 16. I am not against sex education in the form of human biology. I'm not against moral education. What I am against obviously is the teaching of sexual perversion in school.

If I hadn't spent part of the past 11 years of my working life in classrooms and in talking with parents and teachers, as well as pupils, the combined evidence I had just heard from Mrs Riches and Mrs Robson would be likely to damn sex education in my mind. At the very least it would make me highly suspicious of it. Mrs Robson went on to describe what had happened at a meeting in Haringey called to discuss the council's highly controversial decision to adopt positive images of homosexuality. She said:

> I talked at great length to parents from Parents' Rights in Haringey. They have been through the most appalling, absolutely appalling

experience. When they went to speak to their education committee they were spat on, they were struck, they were insulted. They had chewing gum rubbed into their clothes. They were called bigots, fascists, racists, all sorts of things like that simply because they were protesting about the introduction of homosexual education into primary schools. Some of the people in the audience — and we have photographic evidence — were teachers in Haringey schools.

She went on to say:

All around the country there is a great deal of emphasis placed on masturbation. We've been told by children that they find this incredibly embarrassing. I can only presume that the teachers are not properly trained and therefore they express things with gross insensitivity. We're not against teaching the reproductive act. We're against teaching corrupt sexual practices in schools. Inner London has an anti-heterosexist policy now, that they are going to introduce from the nursery up.

Mrs Robson has one point here, certainly. It is quite correct to say that 'teachers are not properly trained', because there is no teacher training college which offers sexuality and relationships as a subject. It has not been considered important enough. While there are no teachers trained in this subject in publicly recognized places of learning like colleges and polytechnics it can always be argued that this is the case. The argument is cynically circular. The subject should not be taught because there are no properly trained teachers. And the reason there are no properly trained teachers is because the subject is not considered important enough for teachers to be trained. At the conclusion of a previous book, *The Ostrich Position* (Allen and Unwin, 1985), in which I discussed sex education as I teach and understand it, I outlined this problem:

While sex education is not a properly formulated subject within school curricula it is not a proper subject and as such is prey to anyone's individual campaign to have it halted. Unless policymakers and curriculum developers choose to accept the subject as important it will continue as it is, a sporadic endeavour undertaken without commitment, and therefore indefensible when attacked. Part of my purpose in writing this book was to move sex education from this untenable position into an area of debate where it could be properly argued and constituted. For unless it is so it will be prone to disappear whenever the going gets rough and in particular will be vulnerable to any individual parents bringing an action against a school or teacher in respect of it. Ironically, while painful for the individuals involved, this may be what is needed to have a fair public debate on the subject.

It is interesting that I should have used the expression '*fair* public debate', for in the middle of this particular public platform I had only just begun to glimpse how *unfair* the contest was. For example Mrs Robson had just made the statement that 'Inner London has an anti-heterosexist policy...from the nursery up.' If this were true it would deeply disturb me. It would be appalling, and would put Mrs Robson and me on the same side of the fence. Somehow I didn't think it *was* true, but given that her statement had been made without documentation or warning, I was not able to refute it. After the programme I rang the ILEA and was told that out of the twelve London boroughs plus the City of London, two, Ealing and Haringey, had adopted the stand of wanting to promote positive images of homosexuality. The others had not. The ILEA spokeswoman went on to say:

> Generally we are concerned with equal opportunities and wish to make sure that homosexuals are not presented in a negative light. We are trying to implement an equal opportunities programme which says that a person should not be discriminated against on the grounds of handicap, race, gender or sexual orientation.

Another problem I had with Mrs Robson's comments concerned the Haringey meeting. I, too, had seen a photograph of this and it showed homosexuals being abused. In the foreground a hetero-sexual man looked as if he was trying to shake the flesh off a homosexual one while the latter refused to retaliate. I had not gone to the meeting but had heard reports that it was stormy and that a great many insults had been hurled around. From these reports I gathered the insults were directed against homosexuals and were, in some cases, vicious. However, I could not dispute what Mrs Robson had said for it is possible that heterosexual as well as homosexual people were struck that night.

But the most extraordinary part of Mrs Robson's allegations was the bit about the pictures of naked women. As I was later to learn, this story is 'misleading' to say the least — and the word is not mine, but the Press Council's. This particular yarn did the rounds in 1986, and began in the *Daily Express* on 8 February as LESSONS IN VICE AT GIRLS' SCHOOL START A STORM. The article read:

> 'A storm blew up last night over lessons in vice at a leading girls' comprehensive school. Angry parents have branded the lessons

at the 1,200 pupil Parliament Hill Girls' School in Highgate, London, "depraved". They are also incensed about 13-year-old girls being told to cut out pictures of naked women as part of a sex equality course. The girls were told to fix men's heads to the torsos, apparently to show them how the media degrade women.'

The school complained to the Press Council. An enquiry was held. On 10 October the Press Council issued a judgement saying that the story was 'significantly inaccurate and seriously misleading' and that the school had not given 'lessons in vice'. Furthermore Maura Healey, the then headmistress of the school, said, 'the source for the exercise of putting a male head on a woman's body was *Good Housekeeping*, and there were no naked women in that magazine'. When the story appeared the newspaper had spoken to only *one* parent who criticized the school: one, mother-of-four Mrs Barbara Robson. That, however, wasn't the end of the matter. A few weeks later on 31 October the *London Standard* carried a story concerning a girl called Myfanwy and complaints about school lessons. The paper quoted Myfanwy, 14, as saying: 'We were told to cut out magazine pictures of naked and semi-naked women in subservient positions and stick men's heads on them...' etc, etc. Myfanwy is the daughter of Mrs Barbara Robson. The acting headmaster of Parliament Hill School, Tony Barnes, wrote a five-page letter to the *Standard* listing 16 points in the article as either untrue, inaccurate or misleading. Only a small part of the letter was published in the paper in November with obviously nothing like the headline prominence of the original story. But by this time the tale itself had gathered the momentum of unstoppable folklore and the *Daily Express* decided to wheel it out again. Under the heading of A MAJOR EXPRESS INVESTIGATION, the paper claimed to 'expose the left's grip on the minds of vulnerable children'. It trotted out a certain story about a mother and daughter's fight to stop such terrible practice and the story was, of course, about girls being asked to cut out pictures of near-naked women, etc. The mother and daughter were of course Mrs Robson and Myfanwy. I became aware of all this when, a few weeks after *You the Jury*, I tuned into Granada's *What the papers say* just at the point where Paul Foot was mentioning something about fixing heads on the torsos of naked women. It was only by chance that I hadn't gone to a meeting that night and had tuned in, more by fluke than by design. I am grateful to Paul Foot and Granada for supplying me with a transcript of the programme from which I have quoted these details.

As the programme continued I began wondering why at the time Norman Tebbit had got it in for the BBC and not the *Daily Express*, or the *Standard* for that matter, and by the end of the programme Mr Foot had given the answer. In reviewing the papers for BBC radio in Manchester, Mr Tebbit had praised the *Express* for what he called its 'first class campaign to expose left-wing authorities which subvert the minds of children.' Ah, well.

Unfortunately, of course, I didn't know all of this when Michael Pipes came to the microphone in *You the Jury*, and it was difficult to make inroads into what had been presented. I was beginning to see that I had somehow to prove the 'evidence' presented as wrong, but how could I with no documents to hand? My original intention had been, simply, to show that sex education as I have taught it, and as Michael Pipes has both taught and supervised it in his school, and as Anna Raeburn has endorsed in so many ways, was sane, necessary and carried out with care and understanding. That hadn't seemed an impossible task. Now it did seem so. But it still seemed to me that I had to try to give people some insight into what proper sex education is. So I asked Michael Pipes his reasons for teaching sex education and for having a programme in his school, and he spoke of the necessity of combating harmful influences in society by arming young people with knowledge. He also spoke about respecting young people's vulnerability. In answer to the question of whether or not parents should have the final say about sex education in schools he answered:

> My wife is the head of a nursery school and, sadly, three- to five-year-olds are seeing at home the sorts of videos that you wouldn't wish your child to see, nor would I mine. The feedback I get from parents is that they are very happy I'm tackling these sensitive and difficult areas with their children. Children don't easily talk about the intimacies of sex or about the mechanics of sex with their parents.

Peter Bruinvels then asked: 'How are you going to *police* the syllabus?' and then further questioned: 'How are you going to *police* it properly to make sure that what you want to see will actually happen?' When asked a further question about 'the teaching of' homosexuality, Michael Pipes concluded:

> I should be very unhappy to think that any member of my staff was doing anything other than that which is normal and down the middle. But they'll get sidetracked into these various branch lines and when they get sidetracked they've got to be bold enough,

brave enough and balanced enough to be able to cope with those questions honestly when they arise.

When I brought Anna Raeburn forward, she emphasized the importance of education in sexuality because of its psychological value:

> I think sex education contributes to emotional health because it is very wrong to deny children or any person the facility and wherewithal to deal with the rest of the universe. And if you deny them that which they can clearly see around them you cause them great pain and great suffering to no good.

When asked what she felt really depraved and corrupted children she said:

> To be denied the possibility of discussing with any human soul that which you need to know: to be cast into the darkness we define as loneliness and like to think that very few people suffer from. Children are essentially lonely and we try to draw them into a real, warm world by offering them all the help and all the love we can give them.

I asked her why she thought people were so frightened of sex education, and she said in a voice which won applause from an audience which obviously warmed to her:

> Because it is an enormous responsibility, and like everything else we have to do with children it is a walk on the water every single time. You may do your very best but you will have no guarantee until much later that you have sown the right seeds.

I finally asked her what she thought the family's responsibility to the child was. She replied:

> To arm the child. To arm the child with love and knowledge and the ability to ask questions, with standards which everyone can respect but which are not narrow; which are generous. And to make it possible for the child to go out into the world and deal with the structures that exist and maintain himself or herself as a person.

Following this, Peter Bruinvels' first question was: 'At what age do you think children should be taught about sex and *perversion*?' (My italic.) Anna Raeburn — perhaps, in retrospect, mistakenly

— ignored this calculated and cynical link of 'sex and perversions' and began: 'I think children start to amass information about people instinctually and naturally from a very much earlier age than makes many adults comfortable...' Mr Bruinvels twice interrupted during her answer and at the end of his questioning slipped in a comment of his own. 'Child abuse is on the increase,' he said, darkly — the implication being of course that it is sex education which causes child abuse. As we have seen before, Mrs Riches had also tried this one, and it is in my view a confusing distortion. Since it is *parents* who abuse *children*, and the parents of today's children did not receive the kind of sex education we are discussing, how can the sex education of today's children bring about an increase in present child abuse? If anything, it will bring about a decrease, for if children are allowed to be aware and respectful of their own sexuality, alarm bells are more likely to ring if a parent or another adult molests them. I cannot believe that neither Mr Bruinvels nor Mrs Riches understands that in cases of incest and child abuse it is the *adult* who is the culprit and not the child.

During his summing up, which followed his comment about child abuse, Mr Bruinvels included the following statements:

> It's quite clear to me that tomorrow's pupils are liable to be corrupted and that undoubtedly a large majority of parents believe that sex is so precious it should be kept within marriage... Sex education as presently practised is a mass of misinformation, misrepresentation and *outright fraud*. Sex education conceals far more than it reveals. There's not a shred of evidence that sex instruction [sic] reduces the number of unwanted pregnancies among teenagers, nor the number of abortions, nor the spread of disease. (My italic.)

He concluded with this:

> The definition of corrupt in the Oxford dictionary says 'rotten, tainted with vice or sin, depraved, influenced by bribery.' Well, it's not bribery we're discussing, but we are discussing tomorrow's adults. The curriculum has never been properly agreed. Teachers are not totally trained and parents, I believe, must now decide whether and by whom sex education should be taught. It's a private matter. The wrong books and the wrong teachers will corrupt and deprave.

When I agreed to go on *You the Jury* I decided not to react to the kind of statements I had already noticed Mr Bruinvels making in the press. I thought it would be better to show through my own experience the benefits of sex education. Maybe I was wrong. The hectoring tones adopted by the movers of the debate had a forcefulness to them that gave them the power of making themselves sound convincing. Moreover they had mixed together in a potent brew the reasonable-sounding with the downright incorrect. For example, 'The curriculum has never been properly agreed. Teachers are not totally trained' is not only a reasonable objection, but also a truthful comment. However, 'There's not a shred of evidence that sex instruction reduces the number of unwanted pregnancies' is simply untrue. There is far more than 'a shred' of evidence to show that sex education reduces unwanted pregnancies — in fact there is a great deal of it. Much of it is contained in the Guttmacher Report, an international survey which shows that countries with more open attitudes towards sex education and contraception have lower teenage pregnancy rates. Other studies done in this country by people like Dr Judith Bury have shown the same thing. Had Mr Bruinvels done any research into this area he need not have looked far to find that the evidence we have points to sex education reducing teenage pregnancy. Anyone is at liberty to disagree with the evidence, but it runs contrary to known facts to say that it doesn't exist.

As to the business of teachers not being properly trained, this is certainly true, and people like myself have been urging that an agreed curriculum and teacher training in this subject be thought out and instigated. People of the Moral Right have fought hard against this idea because they have argued sex education is a family responsibility. So far their persuasion has been the greater. They argue against a full curriculum in schools, and the pressure of their arguments has been such that no-one has taken teacher training seriously in this. By preventing the teaching of the subject they therefore prevent the training of the teachers — and then argue on a public platform that teachers *are not* trained!

Mr Bruinvels' comments about sex education as 'a mass of misinformation, misrepresentation and outright fraud' I had to take personally, because he did not refer to *some* sex education, but to sex education generally. As one of the main practitioners of sex education, with more than a decade's experience of working with thousands of pupils and many staff, to have this work called 'outright fraud' felt deliberately offensive, dishonest and hurtful. My own summing up therefore was somewhat clouded by this. I felt I had to say that I did not practise fraud. I said I was horrified by the catalogue of awful things I had heard, none of which constituted sex education as I had seen it practised and know it to be from my own experience. I argued further that the intimate details and fears about puberty and sexuality generally were things few parents were comfortable discussing with teenagers, that young people must learn about sexuality safely, and that school was an ideal situation for this learning to take place.

At the end of the debate the studio audience voted with buzzers. They had also voted at the beginning of the debate when the motion was first put, so it was possible to see what difference the presented arguments had made to people's opinions.

Mr Bruinvels won there, for although the majority voted against him to begin with and still voted against his motion at the end he had increased his share of 'supporters' by eight per cent and I had increased my share by only two. So the motion was initially 'defeated' by the audience and again defeated at the end, but by a narrower vote. Peter Bruinvels' arguments had therefore been more effective than mine in persuading people to his cause.

CHAPTER SEVEN

Pornography and perfection

At the end of *You the Jury*, just before the final vote was taken, a woman from the audience had a query. She said that she had heard about two different kinds of sex education and wanted to know if she could vote on what kind of sex education she agreed with instead of the motion itself. Understandably the chairman couldn't allow this, and it may have been because of this confusion that Peter Bruinvels picked up some of the supporters he did. For *his* description of sex education could not be condoned by anyone, and because of its sensationalist content, it was obviously more graphic than mine. Since sex education is such a varied and complex subject, dealing as it does with the full range of human emotions, and with many differing attitudes, it is difficult to describe succinctly. The point, however, is not that there are two different kinds of sex education, any more than there are two different kinds of basic biology, basic law or driving instructions. There is the problem that a full curriculum for sex education has never been agreed and therefore its correct practice cannot be monitored because it has not been laid down. The Department of Education and Science has, however, begun to draw up guidelines for it, and a curriculum to follow this will depend on the amount of pressure politicians, educators and parents are able to exert. At the moment the pressure from the Moral Right not to have a full programme of sex education has been effective in keeping the subject tentative and tenuous. But just as road safety training works with clearly defined principles and objectives so does sex education. It is possible to teach any subject well or badly, but a subject itself is not banned simply because some teachers make a poor job of it. The week before the 1986 Education Debate the headmaster of a primary school was jailed for gross indecency and indecent assault on pupils aged eight and nine. His practice had actually corrupted and depraved young children, but no-one called for the banning of either headmasters or primary schools because of it. If there are examples of sex education being practised badly then the individual teachers should be taken to task, not the subject itself. There have been a number of cases of politicians being proved to have lied or behaved immorally, and whether they be Anthony Eden over Suez, President Reagan over arms to Iran, or Cecil Parkinson and his extra-marital affair, the essential practice of government continues. One of the essentials of sex education is that it seeks to produce in young people the ability to govern their own lives, feelings and bodies. It seeks to produce individuals whose use of judgement and ability to think and make decisions is their own. It is in this sense a true preparation for adulthood, where these things are in any case expected of us.

When in the spring of 1985 I gave a talk for the British branch of Research on Sex Education (ROSE) at St Bartholomew's Hospital, London. I made this point fully clear to myself for the first time. The conference was on pornography and I was asked to talk about pornography and sex education. In doing so I had to find, like all of the speakers, a working definition of pornography to be arguing from. So I made the distinction that pornography *discourages* an individual's full knowledge of him or herself and that sex education *encourages* this. Pornography is a terrible piece of trickery, because what it actually does is dissuade you from full knowledge of yourself under the guise of doing the opposite. It appears to be sexually explicit and adventurous, and also at first to be sexually exciting, but in the long term pornography actually militates *against* sexual excitement because it is a drug or an addiction. It is like a fix, in that looking at a particular pornographic picture initially excites, but it soon becomes the case that you cannot get aroused without this picture or a substitution for it. What has therefore happened is that your sexual responses have been hooked into a system which they cannot then function without. The man who can only masturbate to pornography or to a pornographic fantasy is an example of this. The face of his ordinary lover does not bring him to orgasm. He has to 'turn on to' the face in the magazine. In the long term pornography therefore reduces the body's and the mind's overall ability to be open to others and to be sensitive to the small and subtle nuances of an ordinary sexual relationship. This stifles growth, and real exploration. If I am hooked on a large bottle of Scotch a day I'm going to find it increasingly difficult to be satisfied by the pleasures of ordinary social drinking and the relationships and affections that go with it. I need the big fix, and that is my tragedy. Pornography produces addiction, and that is why it brings about a loss of personal freedom and a loss of genuine sexual feeling in the long term.

By defining pornography in this way it is easier to sort out the continuing conundrum that the dividing line between what is pornographic and what isn't, is difficult to define. What we then have to work out from all this is what encourages learning, understanding and the ability for development and growth, and what doesn't. As an educator, my concern is in the area not only of learning *now*, but of encouraging that most precious of gifts, the ability to begin a learning process that will continue into adult life, and indeed for the duration of life itself. The old cliché that we learn until the day we die is, unfortunately, too often untrue. For too many of us simply go round and round the same old ground until we die, and are really little the wiser at the end of it all. Given a picture or shown a film, therefore, and asked to work out whether or not it was pornographic I would have these guidelines to work with. Using these criteria I would therefore not judge as pornographic that which increases our understanding of the human body *as it actually is*. A picture of a naked man would not therefore automatically be pornographic, neither would a picture of a naked woman. What could make either of them tend towards the pornographic is complex, but it is usually in direct proportion to the amount of violence attendant or implied, whether offered or submitted to. But in itself a picture of an ordinary naked body facing the camera is not pornographic. Neither would I call pornographic some of the adult education films I have seen which depict real couples making love. The particular films I saw gave straightforward information, and the motive of being educational was clearly evidenced in their making. There was no coyness, titillation or deception about any of them. Yet these films in particular have had a very limited distribution in this country because of the potential uproar they would raise from the Moral Right. In a healthier moral environment I would unreservedly endorse the use of these films for school leavers and sixth-formers, but even given the opportunity I would never use them in the present repressive and hypocritical moral climate because of the clamour of criticism this would bring about.

Having given my own definition of pornography at the conference I therefore argued that there was no place for it in any classroom I went into, except as a subject for discussion. I explained that my duty as a sex educator was to encourage pupils to knowledge of themselves and to encourage them to knowledge of the body. It was this encouragement to knowledge of the body which the Moral Right objected to, probably because they did not know the difference between pornography and education. I therefore made the distinction again: pornography *discourages* knowledge and development, sex education *encourages* this.

There were many members of the national press, from the big magazines and daily newspapers, present at this meeting. I'm pleased that not only was I not quoted *out* of context, but that what articles there were reported what I had to say in a favourable light. In her article on pornography for *Woman's Journal* (September 1986), journalist Yvonne Roberts succinctly defined the difference between pornography and erotica: 'One is masturbatory sex; the other, a celebration of sex.' She echoed my plea that sex education is a defence against such practices as pornography and incest, not an encouragement of them. However, were I to say that one of my aims in working with young people is to encourage them to celebrate of sex I would again be in much difficulty with the Moral Right, for celebration is not a word they enjoy. I find this anomaly a particular problem because the Moral Right draws much of its evidence for morality from the scriptures, and my own understanding of a scriptural interpretation of the body is that it is a temple. It is the house of home of the mind and spirit and is to be valued, tended and celebrated.

The other thing I do by introducing young people to the wherewithal for self-government is to bring up another dilemma surrounding the concept of ownership and children. As I have earlier quoted Madeleine Colvin as saying (Ch.2), there is no legal precedent for assuming this ownership exists. *Custody* is certainly recognized, but the vexing question of ownership is not actually legally approved. This seems reasonable, for while a child is born to and taken care of by parents who are the child's guardians and custodians, to call parents 'owners' of children is to deny deep spiritual values. These values prize the individual soul and are concomitant with deep educational and social values which recognize that each person is unique and is so *from birth*, not simply from some arbitrarily chosen age such as 16 or 18. But some parents have taken up the cudgels of ownership, and if a letter in the *Guardian* on 16 August 1986 is anything to go by, Peter Bruinvels is one of them. After going through the usual circular argument that 'Teachers in sex education have no real curriculum or experience in teaching sex education, and neither do the inspectors and head teachers', etc (and there are an awful lot of Conservative MPs who have got together to make sure this vicious circle remains true), Mr Bruinvels' letter becomes much more worrying. It contains the statement that 'all parents should be allowed to decide when, in their child's life, sex education should be given and by whom' and goes on the say: 'It is essentially a private matter and *the inherent right of each parent to instruct their child as they think fit*' (my italic). If this were the case, and fortunately it most certainly isn't, it would be monstrous, for if parents could 'instruct' children by *right* this would legalize incest for a start. The day there is such a person as the perfect parent, an inherent *right* might be considered. Heaven knows, it isn't morally, practically or spiritually tenable in a world where politicians lie, powerful people commit acts of treason and terrorism, and where all of us somewhere in our hearts are human enough to have reasonable doubts about ourselves and *no* doubts whatever about our ever-present fallibility. There can never be a perfect parent or a perfect child and it is the search for this impossibility which is in itself a kind of pornography, as is the search or need for a perfect, flawless body. It is a denial of the ordinary and the real, and it nails the souls of ordinary, individual children to the crucifixes of our ignorance and pride.

I wrote to Mr Bruinvels around this time, leading up to the Education Debate, about his campaign to allow parents to have the right to withdraw their children from sex education classes. In an interview earlier on in the year, Chris Patten, then Parliamentary Undersecretary of State for Education and Science, had given his support to sex education within a moral framework. It seemed at first as if Mr Baker would follow this initiative, and this was indeed a hopeful sign. As this became a cause for public discussion Mr Bruinvels led a group of Conservative MPs in opposition to it. Whatever the content of school sex education suggested by the Government, he wanted parents to have the right to withdraw their children. Since I thought this was damaging to individual children and an undermining of sex education I wrote identical letters to Mr Bruinvels, all the party leaders, and the education spokespeople, laying out succinctly my concerns and my arguments. I received replies from everyone except Mr Bruinvels and Mr Baker. After *You the Jury*, when the participants gathered for a drink, I asked Mr Bruinvels why he hadn't replied to me and he explained that he'd received about 2,000 letters in support of his campaign and hadn't yet had the time to reply to all of them. I asked him how he knew all the letters were ones of support since mine had been a plea to him to reconsider his position, and he had nothing to say. However, Mr Bruinvels did eventually send a reply (if one can so describe it) to my letter, three months after it was written. This 'reply' began as follows:

> THE RECENT SEX EDUCATION DEBATE: I must apologize for
> not having written earlier to thank you very sincerely for your
> support, prayers and letter of encouragement, prior to the above
> debate on Tuesday, 21 October. I have been overwhelmed and
> encouraged by the huge number of letters and the very caring
> message included in them. There can be no doubt in my mind,
> that all responsible parents were genuinely concerned by the kind
> of sex education already being taught, or likely to be taught, in
> our schools.
>
> In the old days, sex education was not on the curriculum and
> instead our children received a very modest lesson in biology and
> sometimes, the human reproduction system. Many schools are
> run by left wing councils who have changed all that and positively
> promote homosexuality, at the expense of normal decent family
> and loving relationships. The teachers' personal prejudices are
> certainly being promoted in the classroom, with homosexuality
> being taught as normal and heterosexual relations being *positively*
> discouraged.
>
> In my Amendment which, as you know, I forced to a vote, I
> sought to give all parents the *absolute* statutory right to withdraw
> their child from any sex education to which they object...'

And so it went on. I don't quite know how to respond to a man
who thanks me for supporting him when I didn't. It becomes
transparently obvious from this, however, that it is possible other
letters to Mr Bruinvels also opposed his stand, and he didn't have
the time to read those either. I certainly do not accept that he
has the support he claims to have. What I do accept is that he
has an authority problem with the chief inspector who lives in
his heart. Three times during *You the Jury* he used the word 'police',
asking how this education was to be 'policed'. He also used words
like 'instruction' and phrases like 'absolute statutory right' in
talking about parents' relationships with children when children
are not police cadets and parents are not in uniform.

I also had a talk with both Mrs Riches and Mrs Robson after
the programme, and Mrs Riches commented that I use 'swear
words' in the classroom. I had to say that this was true, because
it is. I *do* use 'swear words' in the classroom, or at least I illustrate
the use of them, for it is the unfortunate case that most of them
are related to sexuality or body functions. In discussing attitudes
to sexuality I ask pupils to consider this. Many young people,
as well as adults, use certain 'four-letter words', and rather than
have these simmering below the surface I bring them out into

the open. Certainly no young person *learns* this language from me, but by discussing the words sensibly my aim is to make the continuing use of them less prevalent. The best illustration I can give of the safety and necessity of this work comes not from a school, but from speaking with a very young friend who had a problem. This friend, a child of eight, let's call her Mary, was having terrible difficulties at school, having previously been happy and achieving well. Her mother found out she was being teased a great deal by some other children in her class who had set against her in such a determined way that Mary didn't want to go to school any more. When I went to visit her one Saturday afternoon she told me this in her own words and was near to tears when she said that the other children called her 'horrible names'. She didn't want to tell me what the names were and hadn't told her mother or her teacher. Since this had been going on for a few weeks by this time, it had obviously gone past a worrying phase or interlude. These things can happen in playgrounds, and are in fact an important part of learning about being human, but they usually pass quickly. This hadn't and Mary had changed from being a child who bounced along to school and loved drawing, writing, playing and especially talking, into a listless, unhappy person. Knowing the power of language, and remembering from my own childhood how words can quite literally haunt you, I thought Mary's problem was that she had let the words affect her so deeply that they were continuing to hurt her after the children who had said them had forgotten the reason for doing so. These 'horrible things' that she couldn't speak were festering inside Mary like unattended wounds, and until they were cauterized by daylight and discussion they would continue to damage her inside. So gently I told Mary that it was important that she tell me what the words were. At this she wriggled away and crouched in a corner of the settee with her head hanging down. Although I found it difficult to do I gently insisted: 'You don't have to say the words if you can't. You can write them down if you like, or paint pictures of them and you can help me work out what they are.' This improved matters a little and she got some pencils and paper as I asked, and came and sat cuddled up to me again. I continued to talk to her gently: 'People who use bad words are being very silly, and they are trying to hurt you. But it's important for you to understand that the words by themselves can't hurt you. That's why you have to learn to say them. If you keep them inside you then they will carry on hurting you, and if you give them to me, or to mummy, then we can take the nasty words away from you and they won't keep on hurting you all the time.' She said 'But I can't say them, they're horrible,' in a low, barely audible voice, and I carried on insisting until she eventually started to write the words, or at least spell them. One of them, predictably, began with the letter 'F' and had three other letters. Another began with the letter 'P' and also had three other letters. She eventually wrote them down and they spelled: 'Fuck off' and 'Piss off'. So I quietly and slowly said the words 'Fuck off' and 'Piss off' a few times just to get her used to the fact that the words *could* be used without hurting her, or in fact being intended to hurt her. The the rest of the things slowly came out.

On talking with Mary's mother it turned out that Mary had been off from school for a day or two because things had got so bad, and talks with the teacher and so on had so far failed to resolve matters. As an only child, Mary is somewhat prone to teasing, so she has to find, with help, her own way of retaliating. But school has always been a joy to her before. Anyway, before leaving that day, Mary was back on form. The unexpectedly morose child who had greeted me at the door had resumed being a talkative, energetic and physically demonstrative person. School improved. Quite simply we had taken the words' capacity for damage and defused them. No-one sensible who had witnessed this could have misinterpreted the use of the words, the intention, or the result. But I'm beginning to understand how certain people try to capitalize on such an approach. They can quite easily say things like: 'Do you know she teaches primary school children swear words. She sits children on her knee and says four-letter words to them and she gets children to write down these four-letter words. Isn't it disgusting?'

Were I to take part in a programme like *You the Jury* again, I would ask for material quoted from to be fully documented, and given a few hours ahead of time to all the people taking part. That way one could be either more sure of its authenticity or in a better position to refute it. The arguments surrounding and supporting the material should be the real test of either side's ability to persuade the audience to its cause — that, and sincerely held views devoid of hysterical or improper supports. For if all parties in this *You the Jury* debate had acted in this way, then the arguments would have been so much more constructive. I suspect the proposing side in this case were actually trying to say: 'We are alarmed about what is happening to children generally, our own and other people's. We suspect that unsound and politically motivated sex education is causing grievous damage and will have far-reaching repercussions. For example can you explain to us why you use swear words in classrooms and what good can possibly be achieved from this.' Had they conducted the debate in such a way, it would have been possible to explain and illuminate. On the subject of Ealing's and Haringey's stand I would have said that I do not support it at all. I, in turn, would have asked them if they thought knowledge of the body was in itself harmful and if so why, and we might all have ended up in a better, a real position to help children. As it *actually* ended, they have filled me with mistrust, and we go our separate ways fighting for opposite things, both supposedly for the common good.

CHAPTER EIGHT
The immoral minority

I ought not to be surprised any more at some of the things which are done in the name or under the guise of being 'good for children'. Too many people lie, cheat and enhance their personal status — a tragedy when it comes to young people. For much of the work done with, and many of the pronouncements made about, young people you require no qualifications, and though this is not necessarily bad, the world of children does attract a large number of adults who think that looking after children is child's play. This happens at both ends of the age spectrum. There is the youth worker I mentioned earlier who was working mainly with 14 to 18-year-olds. Among workers with younger children a survey produced in August 1986 showed that most of the staff who supervise local authority play schemes during school holidays are not qualified. The research, carried out by Play Board, an organization set up by the Government in 1983, showed that most of the 4,000 staff on the scheme had no qualifications beyond those they left school with. 84 per cent of local authorities responded to the survey. Out of approximately 4,000 staff employed on the play schemes just 63 had a playwork certificate, only *two* had a senior certificate, 60 had a playwork diploma and 37 had various other playwork qualifications.

I was once approached by a woman who, with no relevant qualifications, wanted to set up a service for young people. She was a caring woman, but not a very astute one. For behaving unprofessionally with a client she had been dismissed from one agency helping adults, and she rang me to say she wanted to set up a phone-in service for teenagers and would I help with staff training. I read the material she sent and called her back to say that if the staff were volunteers and not specialists they would need more than just an afternoon's work with me. She listened politely as I explained that working with young people was a potentially dangerous thing to do and it needed proper training and a lot of skill. I said that it was possible when trying to give reassurance, especially over the phone, to make things worse. I cited the example of a woman teacher who had told a 15-year-old girl in answer to her question that 'yes, incest was illegal and you could go to prison for it.' What she didn't explain at the time was that it was the adult who could go to prison for it, not the child. It was some weeks before this teacher realized that the girl assumed it was the teenager herself who would be imprisoned, not her father. I explained to the woman on the phone that I myself still made mistakes with language, some of which I was alert enough to rectify and some of which pupils themselves put right, but that it really was a highly complex business. It required understanding of the code some frightened teenagers speak in, alertness to innuendo, and great mental agility. She was obviously displeased to hear all this and said she would ring back, which of course she never did. It was therefore more of a shock than a surprise to read in a local paper some months later that this woman had gone ahead and set up her agency, staffed by volunteers. She was quoted in the paper and on television and made many general pronouncements about teenagers.

In working with children, all too often specialist skill is regarded as unnecessary. All kinds of people may dabble in working with toddlers who would not be allowed, without training, anywhere near the inside of an intricate watch, a personal computer or the workings of a robot. They would certainly not be allowed anywhere near the vaults of a bank or the hard core of a nuclear reactor system. This lack of professional requirement for working with young, vital, highly complex, fast-developing and incredibly impressionable young human beings may well come about from the fact that *having* babies, or the process of becoming a parent in itself requires no skill or talent. It is also the case that a baby's actual needs are not of much consequence to the market-place. Consumerism has tried to inflict bottled milk and unnecessary furniture on unwary parents, but an infant has no buying capacity of his or her own and generally speaking does not attract a large share of market expenditure and advertising. The process of parenting as one that is mainly outside market forces has therefore been terribly under-valued. It does not attract an income or result in a finished product that is measurable.

While our society has underrated parenthood because it is not a commercial or a professional occupation, the Moral Right seeks to re-mystify it. It wants to give parents back some kind of mystical control or ownership, oddly enough as if the child *were* a product with a finite personality and the possibility of set attitudes, and somewhat as if the parents were the mould and the child the setting jelly. In the lead-up to the Education Debate, 'It's a parent's job' rang infuriatingly in my ears many times. I say 'infuriatingly' because my personal experience and reading tells me that the vast majority of parents don't want the awkward job of being sex educators themselves. They are therefore on the whole grateful that schools do this subject (where schools do) and relieved not to have to handle questions they can't answer. In fact most parents have believed for a few years that schools *are* doing sex education. With all the publicity given to the subject this is not a surprising misapprehension. While parents believe this and schools still have no established curricula, hundreds of thousands of young people are emerging into adulthood with practically no information from either home or school. They do have *some* information, and this is from the kinds of places and publications whose purpose is to capitalize on sexual need and ignorance.

Knowing this, I was pleased to be asked by Thames Television to help make a half-hour documentary programme on sex education for the *This Week* series, which was broadcast on Thursday, 16 October, 1986, the week before the Education Debate. So much had already been said by this time by people like Mr Bruinvels that it was difficult to find ways out of entrenched positions. The whole argument about it being 'a parent's job' was, as far as I was concerned, an old one which had been lost both academically and in practice at the beginning of the eighties. So, in discussing the programme we decided that the problem of whether or not parents *should* give sex education was not one we should tackle. However, since the subject had been brought up again, what could be illustrated was the extent to which parents *were able* to tackle the subject. What we could try to do was see if we could find a format in which it was possible to examine parents' ability to speak about sexuality with their children. We resolved the problem of setting about this in the following way: I explained that as part of my work with pupils I try to leave the last hour of our time together free for 'anonymous questions'. During this time I ask pupils to write down on pieces of paper questions they would like to ask or topics they would like discussed. I then put all the pieces of paper in something like a cardboard box, pick them out one at a time, read them, and answer them. If the question is a complicated one we sometimes answer it together as a group. The questions are anonymous because I don't know anyone's handwriting and I take them away with me afterwards so no pupils may recognize each other's writing. This way of working gives shy people the opportunity to ask questions without feeling embarrassed and it increases the general pool of knowledge and understanding among the group. It also goes towards creating a high level of tolerance and concern. My own respect for and handling of the questions is also an example of how to overcome difficult situations and benefit from them, and I've had very few 'joke' questions from doing this exercise. (Once when there were two 'joke' questions in a bundle of about twenty, the 14-year-olds I was working with were so engrossed by the real ones that they told me which the joke ones were! As I finished reading the first a girl said 'Oh, that's a joke one, Miss. Ignore that. Please read the next one 'cos we haven't got much time before the end of the lesson.')

From talking with the programme's producer and presenter about this work the idea for the programme began to evolve. What is important about these kinds of questions from young people, or at least this manner of asking them, is that pupils may then ask what they really want to know about. Asking something which makes you seem either ignorant or prurient is not easy, so often young people don't ask what they *really* want to know but what they think you want them to know. What we could do on the programme therefore would be to film this process of teenagers writing down their questions. We could then get some parents from the school, (although not the parents of the pupils who had asked the questions), read the questions out to them, and see if they were able to answer them. It would show how easy or difficult it is both factually and emotionally to answer the questions children actually ask, rather than the ones we think they ask. This all took quite a bit of arranging with the school, pupils, local authorities and with volunteer parents themselves. Eventually I worked with a group of 16-year-olds for the afternoon, on film, and asked for written questions at the end in the normal way. At this stage pupils obviously knew they were 'on television' but didn't know what was going to be done with these questions. We decided not to tell them initially in case any of them were tempted to ask particularly difficult questions to try to catch parents out. We really wanted questions in as 'normal' a setting as possible. I answered the questions with the pupils myself, and then told them what the questions were for. This gave any of them the option of withdrawing their questions. They had also been allowed to ask as many questions as they liked, so some had asked more than one. After this was done the pupils went home and 11 parents came into school, having been told what they would be asked to do, and had the questions read to them. It must be said at the outset that these parents were very brave. They agreed to come on the show knowing that they would have to answer questions in front of cameras, and when you consider that the people who allowed themselves to be persuaded into volunteering were probably better at answering questions than the many who refused, what transpired was salutary. These were the questions:

1. How is it that there is only a pill for women and not for men?
2. What actually happens when an abortion takes place?
3. Would you recommend the Pill as being the best form of contraception?
4. When exactly is the safe period?
5. Why is it that although homosexuality is discussed it is only the ins and outs and not the feelings behind it?
6. Talk more about a woman's orgasm. What exactly is it?
7. Do you think having sex before you are over 16 is inadvisable or someone asking someone under 16 to have sexual intercourse?
8. Masturbation. Can love come straight away?
9. Social diseases — would regular check-ups be necessary if you were having sex? Contraception — what is the safest?
10. How about discussing why homosexuality is accepted as abnormal and heterosexuality as normal. Why is 16 the minimum age of sexual intercourse?
11. Why do you think that sensitive males are often branded as homosexual?
12. Who decides what contraceptives can be legally marketed in Britain and any availability rules?
13. Would you discuss masturbation and VD. How do men feel about abortion?
14. Can we learn more about diseases? How a woman feels about sex
15. Is it morally correct for a 15-year-old to have sex with a 19-year-old?
16. Would you discuss the age of consent. Should it be lowered or made higher?
17. Do females masturbate as much as men, if at all? Do men feel as strongly about abortion?
18. Is there one method of contraception which is said to be safer and more practical?

This film was made in October 1986 at a time when the AIDS crisis was gathering pace and when certain press coverage of the disease had already approached the saturation point of hysteria. It was shot at a time when the Government was targeting millions of pounds to be spent on public service advertising to alert people to the dangers and the realities of AIDS. Yet the word AIDS was not mentioned at all, before, during or after filming with these parents. In fact in answers to the questions about social diseases no sexually transmitted disease whatsoever was mentioned, and two people in answer to the questions about the necessity for regular check-ups actually said categorically that no, they weren't necessary. No-one mentioned cancer of the cervix which, while it is not a social disease *per se*, is increasing among young women who are sexually active. It can be developed by having only one sexual partner, which is why clinics which specialize in giving contraception to younger women ask that a smear be done within a year of a woman first having intercourse. I mentioned the latter point on the screen, and mention all of these points here not to be critical of the parents who so kindly and bravely took part in this programme, but to illustrate the dangers to young people. In the straightforward question about the 'safe period' there was not a single parent out of the 11 who knew when it was. Many said that there wasn't one, and many also gave the *opposite* of the safe period, saying it was about 10 days after a period had stopped. In the course of talking about the Pill, the safe period and contraception generally, two of the men gave the highly personal information that they had had vasectomies so that contraception didn't really apply to them or their wives any more. The group of parents worked extremely hard and talked the questions over amongst themselves, yet still managed to try to discuss or describe a female orgasm without once mentioning the clitoris. One or two of the questions they clearly misunderstood and occasionally had to say 'I haven't a clue' in reply. At the end of the questions one parent said: 'I think it's very difficult to answer these sorts of questions... I would think that they could be answered much better in a classroom, by a teacher.'

For the concluding part of the filming for this programme, reporter Trevor Philips interviewed the Secretary of State for Education, but without showing him what had been filmed so far. With this last piece of film under his belt he asked Mr Baker, on camera: 'Are you sure parents will have the information and knowledge to guide their children accurately?' The Minister looked incredulous and fell straight into the trap. 'Parents don't have the knowledge about sex education?' he exclaimed. 'I find that a staggering assertion. It's certainly not borne out by my own human observations of life as a family man.' Trap door closes. Following on from a piece of film showing parents struggling to come to grips with children's questions, Mr Baker's comment sounded ridiculous. But, like Mr Bruinvels, he did not appear to want to listen to the actual evidence, from reports, that most parents *cannot* provide adequate sex education and that this is disastrous for young people unless a full programme of sex education takes place in schools. What the vast majority of parents know about the *subject* of sexuality is very little, which I accept as being no more remarkable than most knowing very little about physics or carpentry. What parents should be able to provide is a home with a generally supportive and loving atmosphere. Classrooms are the place for specialist learning and I have always classed sexuality as a specialist subject. I suppose that if Mr Baker were told it was possible to ask 11 parents of teenage children, eight of them women, when the safe period is and not only have none of them answer correctly, but most of them give the time in the menstrual cycle which is *opposite* to this, he would say it was ridiculous invention. If he were also told that these parents were not chosen from a group of less able or disadvantaged people, but rather from a group who were articulate and concerned, I'm not sure what he'd say. But he would probably wriggle out of it.

The argument about whether or not parents should be solely responsible for their children's sex education was actually worked out a long time ago by a long line of parents who have always managed to find this subject impossible to tackle fully. For a while it was felt that the modern parent might be different, and some are, but my overwhelming experience is that parents want the schools to tackle this subject and, as I noted earlier, many believe that schools have been doing so for some time. A briefing prepared by the Policy Studies Institute for the parliamentary debate on sex education showed that 95 per cent of the children interviewed thought that schools should provide sex education. 27 per cent of parents wanted schools to take *sole* responsibility for all aspects of education in sex, the body, contraception and personal relationships, and 96 per cent wanted schools to supplement the parents' role at home in these areas. The report stated:

Parents did not see themselves as good 'sex educators'. They stressed that they did not know how to express themselves and that they or their teenage children were too shy and embarrassed.

Most parents were very critical of the complete inadequacy of their own sex education and, indeed, some had been left in total ignorance of their bodily functions, often to their great distress.

The in-depth study of families concluded that 'if education in sex and personal relationships was left to parents alone, many adolescents would receive no education in these matters'. The report pointed out than most parents were concerned about the way sex is portrayed in videos watched by their children and felt that school discussion would be a far more effective way of counteracting this that parents trying to tackle the subject themselves.

It is evident from all this that to drag the issue back to the stage of argument about whether sex education *should* be given in schools is to be blind to the facts, and to the needs of both parents and children, and is a callous and wilful denial of parental opinion and present reality. It is last decade's argument, not this one's. But there is a further point here that has not been examined and that is the tacit assumption that sex education *ought* to take place in the family. I wonder if this is the case. I have met very few parents who are comfortable discussing sexuality with their teenage sons and daughters. The vast majority have not been comfortable and some have voiced this with the concern that 'it's not right' — that such things should not be tackled at home. An intimate sexual relationship is a private affair, and within the opportunities and constraints provided by family life it's important up to a point that this privacy is kept. In view of this are parents the best people to discuss masturbation, orgasm, wet dreams and vaginal odours with their sons and daughters? One of the things that most strikes you about teenagers when you work with them is their need to distance themselves from their parents' sexuality. A teenager is a developing sexual being and has a great need for his or her privacy. At puberty adolescents need to establish the beginnings of adult independence. They do not at this stage want to be reminded that they were once babies born out of their parents' sexual relationship, which is one of the reasons why adolescents have a strong need to remove themselves from their parents for a while and talk about sexuality with other adults. Another important consideration is that the intimacy and constraints of a family home, and of everyday family life, make it difficult for adolescents to develop sexually without being overlooked. Things like taking much longer in the bathroom are part of a need at this time. And a parent rattling the door handle of making impatient comments may seem much more threatening to a teenager than is intended on the surface. The feeling of being overlooked and of having no privacy is heightened because most homes are not spacious. Parents and teenage children often get under each other's feet. While one hopes that these teenagers have had questions about sex answered honestly at home when they were younger, adolescence may not be the best time to continue the discussion. Which may be why whenever I have asked teenagers whether they would prefer sex education to take place at home or in school they have overwhelmingly answered: 'At school.' The PSI report supports this.

The fact that the seriousness of the AIDS crisis and the Education Debate came together could have had a chastening effect on those opposed to sex education. But it didn't. As the Education Debate approached it became obvious, from reports of speeches and interviews, that the full and proper implications of sexuality and education were not being taken into account. By the time of the Conservative Party Conference a few weeks before the debate, Mr Baker had switched from an opt-out clause to something even more worrying. He suggested leaving the decision about sex education in individual schools in the hands of governing bodies. In other words the subject would only 'happen' in schools where governing bodies chose for it to happen — a large step backwards from Mr Baker's original position set up by Chris Patten, which declared sex education as important and necessary within a moral framework. In order to try to counterbalance the message from the Party Conference I wrote a long article, part of which was published in the *Guardian*, October 1986. The full text ran as follows:

When Government voices start quivering with talk of 'morality' you can be sure that our elected representatives will not be discussing war, poverty, corporate tax evasion or third world famine. They will be discussing sex. And the current furore over sex education had, when it began, all the ingredients of a steamy confrontation: children's moral development, education and parental rights. The Education Secretary, Kenneth Baker, of course knew this, so he decided to adopt what I call the 'ostrich position.' This is the practice of burying your head when things are difficult to tackle and hoping that if you keep it down long enough the problems will miraculously disappear.

Mr Baker's initial problems took the shape of 70 Conservative MPs who rebelled against sex education being taught in schools by saying they wanted to give parents the right to a get-out clause

— i.e. the right to withdraw individual children from classes. As I wrote to Mr Baker at the time, this would have presented a remarkable twist in the genealogy of morals for it would have turned the voice of the 'moral majority' into the practice of the immoral minority. My argument went like this: The regrettably few surveys of parents' views on sex education in schools have shown that the overwhelming majority of parents want schools to help with this subject: a survey by the magazine *Woman*, for example, showed that 90 per cent wanted help. So the Government rebels cannot claim to be speaking for the majority, moral or otherwise, in seeking a parent's veto.

The other factor is to do with children themselves. In the real world children talk with each other in the playground. If one or two children are withdrawn from sex education classes two things will happen. The first is that the withdrawn children will be 'set apart' from the rest of the group and will suffer for this, either in teasing, taunts or by isolation. The second is that they will be told in any case by the rest of the group an informal and possibly inaccurate version of what happened. In other words they will hear in the wrong way. For no matter how good a teacher, the subject of sexuality is so complex that until pupils have been part of sex education for some time there will always be a few who will initially get 'the wrong end of the stick'.

This doesn't even take into account the larger argument of whether it is in fact immoral for parents to deny their children access to education without being monitored to make sure they are doing the job properly themselves.

But to return to my first point, only a minority of parents will withdraw pupils, thus creating isolation for the latter in a climate where head teachers have worked hard to *prevent* segregation and isolation in their schools. That is why I use the phrase 'immoral minority', for I consider it immoral to put children through this unnecessarily unpleasant experience. In 11 years of working mainly with pupils in the classroom and latterly with staff groups, only one child has been withdrawn from one of my classes and both staff and pupils told me of his suffering. In a recent television programme I debated this issue with one of the signatories to the parent's opt-out clause. He was startled when I said the clause was immoral, which I would argue it is if it damages children. What I didn't bring up was the problem of incest. Our available knowledge of incest is still limited but it shows that the numbers of children who are victims of this practice are increasing. At present general figures range from five to ten per cent. And the father who is having an incestuous relationship with his daughter is precisely the father who will keep her from sex education classes — if the Government allows him to. He will do so in case the classes disturb his daughter into confiding her problem and because he fears, correctly, that if sexuality is talked about properly she will begin to question him.

NSPCC reports and figures have shown us for many years that the vast majority of reported damage to children takes place within the family. I really don't know, therefore, why the family unit is thought of as the answer to every child's prayer — or even our own — that children should grow up sound in body, heart and mind. If the Conservative rebels get their way two things will happen. The minority of children withdrawn for 'moral' or religious reasons will suffer the kind of segregation which, in a multi-racial society, many head teachers have fought hard to avoid. The children kept out for immoral reasons will be denied possible help.

What Mr Baker has done now — as he disregards the figures on AIDS, rape and incest as they whistle past his tail feathers — is to make matters even worse than this. He has left the decision about sex education in the hands of school governing bodies. After Mr Baker's speech I spoke with the chairwoman of a school board of governors who said that her colleagues would probably decide to 'leave it up to the parents' and that it would be very difficult for 19 of them to come to a consensus on the subject in any case. So what will happen in effect is that while some school governing bodies will take on the subject of sex education, but give individual parents the right to withdraw, very few will have the confidence to take on the subject without this opt-out clause and most will probably not reach a clear decision.

In other words not only have the rebels, through Mr Baker, won their cause, but they have gone further than that, which for all I know was their original intention. They have managed to get the slow progress of sex education not only stopped, but reversed. This is where the issue goes deeper and is reflected in a word used by Mr Bruinvels in a letter to Mr Baker. He writes: 'I want to see the family unit safeguarded and morality instilled in every child.' The key word is 'instilled'. For education is not a programme of indoctrination but a long process of enquiry which can only be continued into adulthood if a child knows how to think for him/herself. The word 'instil' presumes that teachers are active in putting in and that pupils are passive receivers (and if not passive, to be knocked into shape — in other words, empty vessels). The picture this conjures up for me is one of mental rape. This travesty of education does not allow room for debate, or for individual difference. It also works on the unreal assumption that teachers are always on their toes and never suffering grief, anxiety, conflict, or a change of mind. It sees pupils as never suffering rebellion, boredom or genuine disagreement.

Indeed education in morality is vital and it is crucial therefore that it is education and not indoctrination. At this point parents often ask: 'But how do you educate teenagers without telling them what is right and wrong?' The broad answer is that good teachers seek to *discuss* issues with pupils so that they might [become informed]. A practical example of this goes as follows: a pupil asks if sex before marriage is right or wrong. The teacher says: 'Let's discuss it.' Pupils then say things like: 'It's wrong because a girl gets called names if she does it'; 'Women should be virgins and men don't have to be'; 'You don't know if you're suited to someone if you don't sleep with him first'; 'You could catch VD'; 'Everybody does it these days', and so on. From this a wide-ranging discussion begins and what is remarkable about work like this is the level of engagement involved because pupils are being asked to use their own minds rather than being force-fed other people's attitudes.

I suggest that the morality of education itself is that teachers should not indoctrinate or instil but guide and inform. In educational terms it is therefore immoral to *instruct* a pupil that sex before marriage is right; or wrong. It is people's fear that education is in fact indoctrination which causes so many problems. While there is a fine line between guidance and indoctrination it is, or should be, the purpose of teacher training to produce people who are skilled enough to know the difference. The most obvious example of the complexities and anomalies in our moral lives is the question of killing. We adhere to the maxim 'Thou shalt not kill' yet, through the ages, governments and religious factions have been the biggest instigators of killing known to the human race. Perhaps it has therefore never been in any government's interest to educate children morally, for if this happened the questions asked of us would have no simple answers.

Part of the present dilemma about sex education is in fact based not only on confusion between education and indoctrination but on the fact that there is not a single member of parliament who actually knows what sex education is. I make this extraordinary statement without fear of contradiction because there is at present no standard curriculum for sex education in this country. There is no teacher training college in Britain which offers sexuality or sex education as a subject. While there are Government guidelines for what sex education should look at there are as yet no programmes. The Department of Education and Science has produced a paper on sex education and a document, *Health Education from 5-16*. These begin the work of laying out important guidlelines. While some individual schools have set up schemes of their own these are not yet codified or mandatory. Part of the Government's dilemma, therefore, is that it needs sex education lessons.

In my own work in schools the subject of sex education has included anatomy, morality, history, psychology, legality, changing social needs and attitudes, the family, personal development, hygiene, politics, religion, all birth control techniques (including rhythm and natural family planning methods), individual and collective responsibilities, parentcraft, social skills and exploration of relationships, reassurance, tolerance, trust, knowledge of possible actual physical dysfunction, statistics, and the full range of human emotions and attitudes.

I would argue that teachers need to be specially trained for this highly complex subject. Here you have a chicken-and-egg situation because if specialist teachers are not trained it can always be argued that sex education is not being taught well. Mr Baker has now given the go-ahead for sex education not to be taught at all. It will be a random affair which is a far cry from the Department of Education and Science's own document *Health Education from 5-16* which states: 'Sex education is a crucial part of preparing children for their lives now and in the future'. Mr Baker's stance also [makes a nonsense of an official] letter dated 6 August, 1986 from the Schools Branch of the DES which states 'The Government has made clear its commitment to appropriate sex education in schools as a necessary aspect of preparing pupils for the realities and responsibilities of adult life.'

While politicians make these kinds of about-turns children suffer the present consequences of ignorance and abuse and the future painful knowledge that truth and morality were not always at the heart of decisions made on their behalf.

Since this article was written, it is my opinion that Kenneth Baker has moved education further into the realms of inevitably dangerous schooling.

CHAPTER NINE

The angel on Jacob's ladder

I have changed my mind about some things since I first began teaching in the early 1970s and my teaching has changed accordingly. For example I would now not tolerate, but would take issue with, some of the anti-social behaviour I have worked my way through and round in the past, and which I still see staff working through and round. I would also not overestimate young people's knowledge or underestimate their sensitivity. And remembering this last point, what I have *not* changed my mind about is the problem of personal disclosure. Many young people are at first embarrassed by the idea of a sex education lesson because they fear it will lead to prying into their personal lives and vulnerabilities. I realize that many *adults* view sex education in this way too. They imagine that because sexual intercourse is a private matter, sex education will transgress the boundaries between private and public. Sex education is seen as distasteful because it appears to infringe on the sanctity of what is deeply personal. This is one of the reasons why the *subject* of sexuality as a form of enquiry needs understanding, for sexuality *does* lend itself to objective exploration, and can therefore be treated as a proper subject and not as a series of personal anecdotes or whims.

But understanding and allowing for this fear of personal disclosure, one of the things I now do when I go into a classroom of pupils I have never met before is to say something like the following: 'We are here to discuss sexuality, which means looking at sexual attitudes, general feelings and perhaps general problems. Some of you may be concerned that because we are discussing what you probably call 'sex' that this is personal and private and we shouldn't be talking about it. So before we begin discussing this point I want to let you know that we are not here to reveal anything personal about ourselves, our families or relationships. I want you to know that I won't ask anyone in this classroom a personal question, and I don't expect you to ask me any either.

What we are here for is to see if it is possible to make sense out of sexuality so that it might be helpful to all of us.'

This can be rather a lot for pupils to understand all in one go, especially when you consider that the vast majority of adults they come in contact with do not give them this view of sexuality because they don't have it themselves. We might therefore spend a whole hour working towards understanding sexuality as a general subject rather than sexual intercourse or 'sex' as a private act. Because this is such difficult and necessary work, I might try any of a dozen different approaches to introduce it. I might for example begin: 'The first thing I want to say is that I shan't ask you any personal questions and I shan't expect to be asked any. If we have this as a rule, can anyone tell me how we're going to discuss sexuality and relationships?'

Silence.

So I might ask further: 'Is it possible to discuss the subject of sexuality and personal relationships without revealing personal details about oneself?'

'You can discuss reproduction', says a boy, to murmurs from the others which mean they think he is wrong.

'Quite right', I reply, thanking him. 'I can give you a whole lecture on reproduction without mentioning a single personal thing about myself or anyone else. In fact I could give you a whole lecture on reproduction without even *mentioning* a human being. But I won't.'

They begin to wake up a bit from this and we find out that we are dealing with a *subject*: a subject which has a history, a tradition, a conceptual framework, a changing value-system, and which is affected by and affects other things. What we learn specifically is the difference between the particular and the general, between the personal and the impersonal, and between objective and subjective. This is done through small, simple exercises. I will ask the group for example to make ten *general* comments about the body and then ten made-up *personal* ones. This may produce a sequence such as 'bodies have arms and legs'; 'I have arms and legs'; 'Susan has arms and legs'; 'that body is big; 'John's body is big'. They begin to find this deceptively simple work fascinating perhaps because it is the beginning of important learning. In beginning to understand the difference between subjective and objective, between general and personal, they are initiating the process of acquiring vital skills in relationships and in being able to cope better with their lives. They are also beginning to feel safe. What they are learning is the ability to talk, as they are doing, sensibly and seriously about aspects of life which we keep quiet about. We even discover, for example, that it is possible to discuss emotions objectively, either wholly or partially. We do this through another exercise. I ask them to write down, in a personal form, any emotional problem they care to think of, not necessarily their own, and then ask them to write the same question or problem down in impersonal form. You then end up with things like: 'My boyfriend has left me and I feel really miserable. Can you give me any advice?', which then becomes: 'Can we discuss the hurt that happens when a relationship breaks up'. Or again: 'I feel shy. Is there anything I can do about this?' which becomes: 'Can we discuss how to start relationships and get to know people?'

We continue the exercise in this way, often going into different areas like personal problems generally. They will then write things like: 'I have painful periods. What can I do?', followed by 'Could we discuss menstruation and what causes pain during this time'; or 'I have spots on my face. *Help*', which is transformed into 'Will you talk about skin care and remedies for spots.'

We begin, in this way, to get a feel for the difference between the personal and the impersonal, the subjective and the objective. All of a sudden the language and grammar that they've learned begins to make real, experiential sense as they learn the actual *importance* of being able to distinguish, for example, between personal and impersonal pronouns.

Embarrassment or 'larkiness' in the classroom soon gets dispelled when they realize that they are not going to be exposed either for their ignorance or for anything about their sexual identity or make-up. They learn that you don't have to make yourself vulnerable in order to ask questions in a classroom. They learn that anywhere, at any time, they may ask for information in a straightforward way by saying: 'Will you discuss AIDS with us', or 'What is the efficiency of the Pill?' And they begin to learn that if someone mocks them for not asking a straightforward question, then *that* person probably has considerably more problems than they do.

My task in the classroom is to reassure and enable. Part of the reassurance is to let pupils know that it's possible to discuss unhappy homes without discussing 'my' unhappy home, to discuss fears about sex without discussing 'my' fears, to discuss hurt feelings without discussing 'my' hurt feelings, and so on. This does both reassure and enable, and it takes sexuality and relationships from the personal into the impersonal or objective in the correct way, as a fitting and important subject for rational discussion and enquiry. This enables a girl who is involved in incest for example to learn that this is not only a personal hell visited on her (probably because she thinks she is a bad person) but a bad adult practice that people visit on children from generation to generation because adults have problems, not because children are born wicked. It takes this subject from the personally unmentionable into proper public discussion. In this way the child may learn that everyone's personal anguish or joy, as well as being unique, has a shared place in the sum total of human experience. This kind of possibility for children, of learning that their personal lives are connected to the world generally and to issues in the world, is a very important and benign process. It gives them a place in the world which they can then feel a part of. So often the word 'alienated' is used to describe disaffected youth. It is an apt description of what it feels like not to belong, and often results in self-destructive and anti-social behaviour. Offering young people concretely, through sound education, the chance to learn and understand about 'belonging' helps to make alienation less likely. It is the understanding that their inner worlds have an outer context which enables teenagers to move from selfishness to empathy and care for others, which is what we expect, and need, from them as adults. We often try to demand this with comments like: 'You're not the only one in this house you know. Other people have feelings too.' We want them to understand about being considerate to others, but we try to force this on them rather than leading them to it. In the kind of work I have described in the classroom, pupils are given a concrete way of getting outside their often intense personal preoccupations and are given the transforming power of making general sense out of individual circumstances. In other words they are given the possibility of *meaning*, of discovering purpose and shape and connections between their own lives and the lives of others. This in turn brings about a strong two-way process of encouraging a movement outwards, and also the return inwards. In this way, at the same time as gaining more understanding of the world around them, they will also bring that back to themselves and gain more self-knowledge. A. N. Whitehead himself in *The Aims of Education*, (Williams and Norgate, 1929. Second edition, seventh impression, Ernest Benn, 1970), writes of this two-way process in the following way: 'It is merely a barren game to ascend from the particular to the general, unless afterwards we can reverse the process and descend from the general to the particular, ascending and descending like the angels of Jacob's ladder.'

It is delightful to work with young people in this way and to enable them to discover that they have much more to say than they at first thought. They realize that we may discuss the most 'intimate' of subjects objectively and *not* be more than only slightly embarrassed to begin with. So it is possible for me, as a woman, to discuss female orgasm in an objective manner, explaining where the clitoris is, explaining that every human body is different, and that therefore sensations are found, felt and described differently, that there is no formula for sexuality and relationships, and that this is part of its continuing wonder. The business of making sexuality objective in this way, whilst retaining its humanity and personal relevance, may be the key to explaining to adults how the work may be done well and safely in a classroom. So many times adults shake their heads when I say I discuss sexuality with young people and cannot understand how this can be done without acute embarrassment or possible offence. Not only is it done, where it is allowed, without the school falling down, but it is part of the vital learning which will enable young people to continue growing and developing through their lives. For people who are embarrassed and diffident are not in good positions to cultivate responsibility for themselves and others, and if responsibility is what we want from people, then we won't get it by denying teenagers information and skills which they need. By experiencing what it is to be part of easy discussion, pupils gain positive resources with which to continue their development. For a start, they begin to learn how to *listen*, to themselves as well as others.

I am very often struck by the emotional 'temperature' in a classroom. In a classroom which begins as seeming cold I usually work in a low-key way with the intention of 'warming it up a bit' by raising the tone and temperature. But very often I work the other way round. Many classrooms I've worked in have been 'over busy' at the start. There has been a lot of chit-chat and far too high a level of nervous energy. My intention then is to calm and soothe the climate so that we reduce the pitch and find, after a while, that we're speaking harmoniously together. It is so rewarding to be part of an endeavour, almost like a conductor of an orchestra, where you arrive to general clamour and end up with a group in unison, or in tune, with each other. Sometimes I will make this explicit at the end of the work and say simply that it has been good to see how we have worked together and how well and carefully we have listened to each other and learned. I also sometimes talk with older pupils about naming the unnameable, which is another important aspect of sex education. We learn that there are few of us who have not experienced dreads of some kind or other and that naming the dreads can move us from a position of near paralysis to one of finding the help we need. With sexuality in particular I am struck by how ordinary some of the dreads still are: a salutary reminder that we have *not* produced a generation of young people who don't suffer from or fear things like bad dreams, bad breath, shyness, impotence and ignorance. To add to their repetoire of skills is as important as adding to their repetoire of knowledge, if not more so. The former will enable them to find out on their own and will increase their stature in a way which is not strictly controllable by us. Is that why many of us fear it? It's as if we're afraid of becoming a company of dwarfs among the giants our children might become if allowed to develop fully. Why should this be? What makes us think these giants would be anything but benign and kindly?

The ability to make sexuality objective is a skill it would be unrealistic to expect most parents to have, and yet to some extent this ability is vital for sex education to take place at all, in the home, where both parents' and teenagers' need for privacy must be respected especially. As I quoted Michael Pipes earlier: 'Are parents really the best people to do this subject? Why should we presume they are?' Of the parents who were filmed for the programme described in the last chapter, two of the three men present gave highly personal information about themselves on camera in answer to questions about the Pill and the safe period. They said they had had vasectomies. In the *objective* answering of the questions asked this information would be entirely irrelevant. Within a family it could be extremely perplexing to a teenage son or daughter. For most teenagers, their wish *not* to know about their parents' sexual lives is as pronounced as is most parents' concern to try to control their children's. Therefore being told that a father has had a vasectomy could be highly disturbing to a teenager, especially in answer to a question about contraception. And objectively speaking, vasectomy is not relevant to a young person's life.

If sexuality is viewed *only* as highly personal, instead of as an area of knowledge and enquiry in its own right, one might indeed claim that it does not belong in a classroom. But perhaps the reason most teenagers don't go to parents for help is that they are afraid not only of revealing themselves but of having their *parents* reveal themselves. I'm not sure for example that it would usually be the case that a father or mother could show a teenage son or daughter how to use a condom. Why is it imagined that boys in particular are born with an innate knowledge of how to use one? The AIDS epidemic has made it essential that everyone knows what a condom is, what it does, what its limitations are and how to use it. Many of the boys I have met haven't a clue how to use a condom properly, and a woman who works in a family planning clinic told me recently that the number of calls from young men ringing up to ask advice about condoms has increased dramatically. This brings with it its own horror stories, like the 15-year-old boy who told me that in his all-boys school two male teachers told them how to use sheaths by using a broom handle as a prop. The boy felt particularly squeamish about this, and no wonder! It certainly shows a ridiculous squeamishness on the part of the staff concerned. With the right attitude there is nothing wrong with using the two fingers of one hand as a prop for demonstrating how a sheath is correctly used. I have never had any trouble from doing so.

As it happens, AIDS has transformed the sheath into potentially life-saving equipment, but there is no need to use the tragedy of AIDS to justify full programmes of sex education in schools. What AIDS has done is to throw up moral as well as medical questions which are extremely difficult to answer. As panic buttons have been pushed, moral about-turns have accompanied them. As one Conservative MP has already demanded the legalizing of brothels one could believe for a moment that the illness was not a god-given punishment of homosexuals but an act of divine retribution against the Moral Right. The latter were now having to ask people like myself whom they had scorned as fraudulent and perverse to help communicate a life-or-death message to school children. The people who wanted sex education banished from schools were having to concede its necessity. What is really interesting is that I didn't read any suggestion in all this that information about AIDS be left to parents. I didn't hear anyone say that it wasn't the Government's or the school's concern to try to protect children and young people from AIDS. I presume it was felt, correctly, that it would not be safe to leave this job in the hands of parents.

When asked in interviews about my work in the classroom it is impossible to explain or do justice to it in a few sentences. If I said these days sex education is about saving lives I suppose people would respond to this. But I would hesitate to do so, for sex education has always been about saving lives, that is if it is the *quality* of lives one is concerned about. The argument for not leaving sex education to parents may be made clearer if, because of AIDS, one looks at just a few medical aspects of modern sex education of which you could not reasonably expect parents to have anything like a comprehensive knowledge. To begin with, even keeping up to date medically means reading a fair number of journals. It means having the latest information on research on the Pill in particular and on contraception in general. It means being able to discern the difference between rumour and hard fact. It means knowing of the latest developments in 'surrogate motherhood', being completely up to date with information about diseases like herpes and AIDS, and, very importantly, knowing about the latest research on cervical cancer and its link with genital warts and wart virus infection. One needs to know the latest moves afoot to tighten or repeal the abortion laws and to be abreast of moral and medical issues such as the moves afoot to try to give putative fathers rights to the *foetus in uteri*. And it is most important to be able to relate all this information to attitudes and morals past and present, and to other subjects. For example it was beginning to seem intellectually reasonable in an age of equal rights that putative fathers have a say in whether or not a woman has an abortion. However, when an Oxford student, in the spring of 1987, took a case to the Law Lords to try and prevent his girlfriend having a termination, he lost. Would it *ever* be morally defensible or medically enforceable for a woman to carry on with a pregnancy at the instruction of a man? And can a man claim to be a father when the foetus is still in the womb? What is his proof of paternity? And so on.

And these issues probably constitute less than five per cent of the overall content of sex education. The whole realm of emotions, attitudes, responsibilities is vast, as is the history of sexual practices and attitudes and the differences past and present in cultural, geographical and religious aspects.

Given how much we keep secret, it is hardly surprising that each generation of young people imagines it is *they* who have invented sex. Nor can one be surprised when they imagine their parents never 'do it', and that their grandparents were probably brought about by some unnamed juxtaposition between a goose-berry bush and a convenient stork. The idea that parents should be solely responsible today for proper sex education is completely untenable. Yet the fear of leaving it in the hands of untrained people is an understandable one.

The answer to the dilemma is, surely, to train teachers.

CHAPTER TEN

The predictable pendulum

Education has come such a long way since I left school that it's easy to understand how what goes on in classrooms these days is sometimes incomprehensible to parents. The progress from the Victorian prison which operated on the premiss that children were there to be tattooed with the correct moral pattern, to a modern sixth-form where a teenage boy may write 'I would like to walk barefoot through your hair', has been swift. The negative side of this rapid progress would, for some people, be the rise of such subjects as sex education and personal studies.

The head of sixth at Chase Cross School, Romford, Essex, finds the threat to education takes a different form. Martin Hayes has the following to say about the dangers to and benefits of good education:

The big danger now in schools is machinery, and the relationship between adult and child will be disrupted by this. I think it's necessary for people in general and children in particular to have personal relationships. You've got to have people *taking* with each other. Increasingly, however, machinery in education is talking over. We're talking in the school I work at about computers across the curriculum. And what will that mean? It will mean there will be more contact of pupil with machine and less contact of pupil with teacher. Of course there's a place for all that because computers are a part of our lives, but one mustn't forget the deeply important thing, the value of personal contact.

I get a great deal from the personal contact of teaching, like seeing a pupil grow through a problem. Sometimes they come to you because a parent is too close to the problem, and you put points of view to them that hadn't occurred to them and watch the wheels go round as they go away and think. You're there as only a kind of prompt to their own thought and feeling processes. I find pupils' personal development very satisfying and enjoy seeing them come to terms with sometimes a sexual problem, sometimes a learning one.

The worst thing of all is giving advice, which is what I avoid doing. The danger in doing this is that you're not that person. You're not in his or her head. You only know as much of the situation as he or she has let you know and even then you're interpreting it from a point of view which isn't theirs. To say 'you should do' from this position could be very damaging.

What is true here is that a child's moral development is neither its teachers' nor its parents' direct concern. Moral development is something we must do and find for ourselves, facing issues as they occur to us and being presented with different sides of a moral or ethical issue and being told 'Go away. Think about this from different directions and find your own solution.'

Here the preachy parent is as big a damage to the well-being of society as the preachy teacher, and I'm afraid Mrs Gillick would be as much danger in a classroom as a doctrinaire Marxist. She would just put forward her own point of view. Children are not yours you know. They are not possessions. They are free individuals, and they've got to explore the world in their own way.

And in any case I can't accept these notions of absolute good. Yes, we could agree generally that to be loving is good and to care is good. But if you successfully indoctrinated a child with these how is he to learn the gradations? How is he to learn when it is appropriate to love more or less and how is he to learn about the full experience of caring if he takes it as a fact of life rather than as something which is often a struggle? Where is his individual triumph over his own feelings of despondency?

If schools do get heavily computerized — and it looks as if we're losing the battle against this — we will have a return to Victorian values where the academic curriculum is all that counts and the personal skills side is mainly dealt with completely separately. This is highly dangerous, for it will take the human element out of the academic, and surely we've learned by now that we can't afford to do this. It will also devalue the personal and the social, and therefore people will be of less account. I know I'm fighting a last ditch effort against this separation, but we are in danger of de-humanizing the academic curriculum. Instead we ought to be looking properly at how to integrate personal and social education into the curriculum as a whole, for every teacher should be a teacher of personal and social education. Whether you're a maths or a history teacher you are still a teacher of people and you mustn't forget this. You're not just a teacher of a subject. But the advent of educational technology is going to bring about a big split in the curriculum.

I asked Martin Hayes how he saw the role of parents as a supplement to personal education in school:

No child can tell a parent everything and it varies from child to child what that something is that they can't talk to their parents about. Some children can't talk to their parents about their courses and their learning difficulties. Some can't talk about relationships and others can't talk about appearance and dress.

The same is true of staff members. Some of my pupils can't talk to me. They'll go to a different staff member instead. In particular, children won't come to me if they want an *answer*, because I've got a bit of a reputation in the school for posing questions rather than giving answers.

As for the kinds of questions, they have varied enormously. Lads have come to me because they haven't started to grow facial hair when most of the others in the group have. Girls have come to talk about contraception when perhaps they've tried their mums who have said something like 'What do you want to talk about that for? Don't you realize you shouldn't do that kind of thing till you're married?' And that isn't what the girls have wanted. They have just wanted the chance to talk with somebody close and they may have come to the conclusion themselves at the end of the day they should wait. But they wanted to talk, not to be lectured at.

What I have found is that you can't predict who will come to you, for the very person you thought was tremendously self-assured and had a good relationship with his or her parents will be the one who turns up on your doorstep. You also have to be pretty aware to know how far to take things when a pupil comes, say, to talk about an essay. Let's take a scenario. X has plucked up the courage to come and see you and bowls through the door. He suddenly realizes as he does do that he doesn't want to talk about his problem yet, not to you, and you've got to have the nous to be able to sense this and still allow him to back out. That happens quite frequently, and you have to respect it. The worst thing that happens is when a parent rings up and says: 'Will you have a word with my daughter or son'. And you have to say in the politest possible way 'No'. You have to explain that you're there to help if the pupil comes to you in any case, but you're really only there as a sounding board. This is hard for some parents to take.

When we went on to discuss how he saw the particular role a school plays in people's lives, he said:

Whether they're five years old, ten years old or 93, people have to have their own concerns. Many children want from education the chance to explore their feelings and their attitudes towards each other. Parents will be an obstacle to this happening because they've come up through a different system and have been socialized by it. Employers will find it a problem because they want a shorthand way of judging people, and exam results give you that. However, teachers have to have a measure of autonomy in the classroom. I believe in what I'm doing and people would have to be threatening me with dire things to make me change. I know education should be about personal development, about personal liberation, and anyone who prevented me from teaching in this way would probably make me drop out of the education system. It takes kids a while to get used to the fact that you're not going to be there to give answers but to ask questions, and they don't always initially like this themselves. But I'll give you an example of a girl, let's call her Anne, who did this and ended up doing something I regretted, but had to accept was her own decision.

Anne's relationship with her mother was a very ambivalent one. On the one hand she respected and loved her mother and on the other hand her mother told Anne to do things which were against the lass's inclination. So there was this internal clash. On the one hand she wanted to obey her mum and on the other hand she wanted to be her own person. This problem reccurred in different guises right the way through her sixth year. She had learning difficulties, relationship difficulties and problems with her self-image. The first occasion it was presented to me was when her mum wanted her to be a teacher. Anne didn't want to be a teacher but thought she'd be letting her mum down if she turned her back on a teaching career. Her problem was, who should she please? She didn't express it quite like this, but that was the essence of it.

A little later she fell quite heavily in love with a lad, and although quite a reserved youngster herself the relationship had been going a couple of months and they'd reached a point of talking about a sexual relationship. She'd tried to talk to her mum, but her mum had reacted badly and said things like: 'Who do you think you are, some kind of slut? I'm not prepared to talk to you about this. It's wrong and you know it's wrong. I'm always right and you must listen to me...'

A couple of days later Anne came to tell me about all this. What she wanted initially was some straight facts about birth control. I could give her this, but I knew there was more to it than that. She was still caught in her own mind about whether she should really be entering a sexual relationship at all. Her mother had placed so much guilt on her that even had she disobeyed her mother she would have been carrying even more problems on her shoulders. In the end I asked her if she was quite sure she wanted to go into this sexual relationship and she said that she wasn't at all sure. She said that although she wanted to, and her boyfriend (let's call him John) wanted to, she had to take notice of what her mum said.

So we began to talk about this. Should she listen to her mum or should she live her life for herself? She was really torn. She didn't resolve this right the way through her first year sixth. But at the end of the year she finally made a decision. From my point of view it was a disaster because she decided to leave school. She decided to go against her mother, to begin a sexual relationship with John and to get a job and save up so that they could live somewhere by themselves.

John came and saw me separately at this time. He'd just failed his 'A' levels and had had a disastrous time. But he came to say that now that Anne had made this decision he felt a lot better. He said that their relationship had been really tense and difficult, but that now Anne seemed happier and more relaxed and things were changing rapidly for the better between them. And although Anne left school when she was a very promising student with bags of talent, in one way I was happy for her because she was beginning to live her own life.

When caterpillars turn into butterflies they go through a chrysalis stage and they're shut up in that chrysalis. You might think you're doing them a big favour by cutting them out but if you do that you're going to kill them. All you can do is put them in an environment where they can develop for themselves and turn into butterflies. If you try and do things for them that's the big disaster. I could have given Anne all kinds of advice, but she had to work it through herself. I was just glad to be there when she felt in need of someone to talk to and I was pleased she could pop in the door if she felt like it and cry her heart out and express her frustrations. She knew there was someone there who was not going to condemn, or praise, her for what she was doing, but would just understand and say: 'Well, how are you going to make something out of how you feel?' It took a whole year for her to do that — make something out of how she felt.

You ask me about the forces railing against education as I know it; the forces that want to bring pressure on young people to be what we want them to be. In the end it's the triumph of the human spirit. No matter how much someone tries to lay down for you how you must live your life, in the end the spirit seems to triumph. You can see that spirit throughout history in people's resistance to abominable authority. You do see reactionary forces in society but I believe the human spirit will always triumph, and in some ways that's the only thing that keeps me going — that despite every opposition you have an inside self.

It is to that inside self that I intrinsically address my own work, to the self that is hidden, struggling, and which is more than anything else unique. It seems particularly important that the latter is stressed in all manner of ways at the moment because of the dangers young people are in by not being offered a full grasp of this. The problems of glue-sniffing, drug-taking and pressures to look for short-term kicks rather than long-term gains are strong. And despite this, time and again teenagers are sold short of the ability to be their better selves. Both for the present and for the future they need courage to go against the pressure put upon them to join a gang or run with the pack. It is a brave *adult* who will stand up in a group of people and be the odd one out, and it's asking a great deal of young people that they should do the same. One of the ways to help them towards this and also reduce the power of the gang ethos or peer-group pressure is to work with the idea of uniqueness clearly in mind. If young people really did know, from caring for their own and other people's individuality, that gangs abnegate what is truly human the latter would not flourish. By stressing both individuality and the co-operation which is part of finding and learning about oneself one stresses what is important at a time when muddled thinking and sticking together for its own sake are prevalent. The problem of working in this way is that the effects of doing so are not easily or immediately measurable. They could be, were we interested in developing exam papers which asked questions such as: 'Discuss some current conflicts between individual and social responsibility. Is one more important than the other?'. Or again: 'What is the age of consent? Give reasons for making it higher or lower or for leaving it as it is', and so on.

At the moment the field of personal development or learning to think individually is not part of the mainstream school examination system. Sociology and personal and social education cover aspects of this, and are still not taken seriously in those many schools where they are viewed as non-academic and therefore less important subjects. Yet aside from the skills of literacy and numeracy the ability to think for oneself is above all others crucial. Without it we would be of diminished responsibility and therefore not legally, personally, morally or spiritually accountable. It is the ability to be able to understand the possible consequences of our actions which gives us our ethical dimension. The learning of language, mathematics, geography, carpentry or music does not in itself do this.

In addition to this problem of what is principally important for young people to gain from education, both at home and in school, there are the problems of the kinds of adults who take an interest in young people, their real reasons for doing so, and some of the unexpected results of otherwise apparently good and well-meaning I'm thinking in particular of two important campaigns set up in 1986 to try to help children and teenagers. One was a campaign against drug addiction, with the emphasis on heroin and glue-sniffing. The campaign alerted young people to the dangers of these drugs by illustrating what awful side-effects they had. In an article in the *Guardian* (18 August, 1986) Richard Ives, who works at the National Children's Bureau, explained why some of the media coverage of glue-sniffing was doing more harm than good. He began with a story about the difference between tape-recorded transcripts of young people's experience of glue-sniffing and edited results:

> In the original transcript the young man says: 'Sometimes when I sniffed I felt sick, often I was sick. Then the hallucinations started. They were fantastic. It is the hallucinations that are the real attraction of glue. You are excited beforehand because you never know what is going to come out of the bag. That's why it is best to sniff in a group.'
>
> When the transcript appeared in the magazine it read as follows: 'Sometimes when I sniffed I felt sick. Often I was sick. Then the hallucinations began. It is best to sniff in a group.'

Like everyone else I can understand the reason for the omissions, for to report glue-sniffing as having 'fantastic' experiences attached to it might encourage others to sniff and would be deemed irresponsible journalism. The reporter here, therefore, appears at first sight to be behaving professionally. The problem is that her keeping back of essential elements of the truth has negative results, as Richard Ives goes on to explain, beginning with another example of edited material:

> The young woman's original transcript reads: 'My marriage lasted two years. We had good times. We were both sniffing when we married but at the time that was all part of the fun. I remember once being over the park with 'X' when we were both high. he said he can make something appear out of nothing. I said: "Go on then." He made a whirlwind appear. It was fantastic; even more strange that we could both see it. We often shared the same hallucination. One day we watched a giant frog jump over the house. Another day we saw an elf run across the park. It was so vivid. I still wonder if it had been real. We did not eat in any regular way. You feel apathetic after coming down.'
>
> As published, that section reads: 'My marriage lasted two years. We had good times. We were both sniffing when we were married but at the time that was part of it all. We did not eat in any regular

way. You feel apathetic after coming down from glue, you have no appetite.'

Just about all the amendments erased references to the enjoyment of using solvents and to satisfactory or interesting hallucinations. References to bad hallucinations are reported in full, for example: 'I had bad hallucinations. Once straps whipped me around as I was sitting in a chair, then swords came up through the floor and went right through me. I screamed out in agony. I looked in the glue bag and it was full of blood.' The cumulative effect of all these changes is to alter substantially the meaning of the experience which these two young people had while they were on glue. The journalist responsible may well argue that such alterations were carried out in order to behave in a responsible way. *But the changes make the experience of sniffing, as it is reported in this magazine, totally unintelligible. We have no idea why such apparently articulate youngsters have got involved in it.* (My italic.) It is like describing the experience of consuming alcohol without mentioning the camaraderie of the public house or the pleasantness of alcohol intoxication, while stressing the expense, the danger, and the vomiting. *The sniffers' experience is made to sound so unpleasant we cannot imagine anyone we know indulging in such behaviour, and if we find someone sniffing then our reaction is likely to be an inappropriate one because we have no understanding of their motivation...*(My italic.)

I would agree with this. It is news to me that one can see elves and wonderful frogs as a result of glue-sniffing, and this certainly helps me to see, as I didn't before, the lure of this practice. In the way I work at the moment I make distinctions for young people between what one may call *natural* and *induced* 'highs'. As with the business of pornography, drugs bring about induced pleasures which in the long term militate against natural ones because they detract from your ability to grow. But in order to help young people fight addiction, the more fully accurate descriptions I have of it the better I and they shall be served. Another feature of this understandable but dangerous omission on the part of the journalist is that, as it stands, it could in fact *encourage* glue-sniffing. If only part of the story is told, and is brought forward as evidence for the dangers of glue-sniffing, a potential addict could say 'That's not what it's all about. They've cut out all the best bits. The press always do that. They print what they want. There isn't a word in there about the pictures you see and the magic you can make. They don't want us to do it so they only tell us what they think we should know.' True. And as such it will ring loud messages to be taken up by other young people.

The fact that adults lie, either deliberately or by omission, covers a great variety of sins. And every well-intentioned media lie, or any other kind, makes it more difficult to tell the truth eventually, and to be believed. On this point in particular I'm thinking of the other 1986 campaign, Esther Rantzen's *Childwatch*. I thought it was a step in the right direction that the subject of incest 'came out' in the early 1980s. I was also alarmed at the unscrupulous and pornographic methods used in some of the popular press to describe it. I use the word 'pornographic' because some of the coverage of incest was designed to knock us senseless with sensationalism and therefore render us less capable of real feeling, particularly of compassion. There was no doubt that by 1985 the subject of incest had gone from relative obscurity to near notoriety. By 1987 the storm of Cleveland had shown up the complexities, problems and fiercely divided loyalties this subject can evoke. It was worrying to realize that so soon after the existence of child abuse was beginning to be publicly acknowledged, a case like Cleveland should raise the kinds of antagonistic questioning it did. There's nothing that damages people's ability to care more than overkill. In the case of *Childwatch*, the problem was slightly different. It was the leaving out of one word which caused me concern: not exactly being economical with the truth, but trying to exact from the tragedy just that fraction too much. The word that was left out was 'young'.

The first and final line of defence for an adult accused of incest is to say that the child is lying or making up a story out of his or her imagination, and there is no doubt that in the past adults have been believed in preference to children. We still think of 'adult' as meaning responsible and truthful. In working out whether a child is lying or making up stories there is a rough guideline to help us. It is considered that young children will not lie or make up stories of incest, but that older children might do. That is not, of course, to say that they *will* do. It's just that in presenting evidence, medical knowledge suggests for a court's guidance that the words of a five-year-old be believed. Psychiatric learning tells us that young children do not have the necessary verbal and mental make up and dexterity to invent a story of incest. The *possibility* for doing this increases as the child becomes older and has the wherewithal and the knowledge to invent, although this is not to say that this *actually* happens. The age at which the child changes from being virtually unable to lie about this to having the ability to do so varies, and is in any case difficult to judge. But since it is crucial to have some idea of it the age is presented as approximately eight years. So a child of six is highly unlikely to be lying, but a child of nine may be, as may a child of eleven or twelve. This is the complexity of the issue as we understand it at present. The overall message is obviously to take all reports of incest extremely seriously and to give all children the opportunity to speak. For a child who lies about incest needs help in any case. If these matters are handled wisely, then if a story of incest is false an innocent adult will not be brought to task and a disturbed child will receive proper professional support. On her programme Esther Rantzen took up this point about lying when initially interviewing a child psychologist and it was agreed that young children tend not to lie about these things. Unfortunately she then dropped the word 'young' and this comment afterwards came out as 'children tend not to lie...'. The omission is so important. There will have been many parents and young people watching *Childwatch* who knew this comment of Esther Rantzen's not to be true. This would have discredited in their eyes a programme which was full of heart-rending case histories illustrating the prevalence and the trauma of incest. These need our sympathy and care, and any alienation of these qualities for a small slip of the tongue is a hardening against suffering which we cannot afford. The biggest defence any of us has against being deeply concerned in a world where mass communication brings us so many tragedies is to know that the news is exaggerated or not true, and like the hardening of arteries in the body, the hardening of hearts is extremely dangerous.

One of the many problems I found with the irresponsible section of the press and its coverage of incest was the way it separated adults and children off into 'us' and 'them', again causing an inevitable hardening of hearts against the genuine suffering of both. They (children) were presented as the victims of us (the monster adults). It is the setting up of the idea of two separate breeds. Children and adults are not two separate breeds. Children are young or not-yet-developed adults and adults are or should be developed or grown-up children. It is adults who remember that they were once children and who reconcile themselves to the pains and joys of their childhood who are least likely to damage young people. It is the adults who call the child 'other' and set the child apart from and outside themselves who do damage. They do so because once something is set apart or segregated it becomes less easy to identify with and more easy to 'knock'. While we remember childhood as being integral to us our children will be much safer than if we divide adulthood and childhood into two separate camps.

The correlative of this problem is that created by another group of people who make life difficult for children, and for the rest of us — those who over-identify with young people. As if to do the opposite of separating themselves from childhood they continue it through their own or other people's children. They have learned from looking at their own childhood that to condition children heavily is wrong, and they then make the understandable but potentially disastrous mistake of deciding that all conditioning of any kind is wrong and must cease forthwith. This takes the form of letting young people do as they like, a kind of domestic *laissez-faire*. They therefore fall about laughing when a teenage girl tells a story about some slightly thuggish behaviour she has been involved in, and smile when a teenage son tells of an incident redolent with bad manners. I have come across many examples of this. When it happens with teenagers, it is as though the adult tries to re-live or re-create his or her own adolescence and live it vicariously through others.

Two examples of this occurred a few years ago when I was interviewing both adults and young people in various organizations set up to help teenagers. In one a counsellor was putting away some things in a file when a young girl of about 15 came in. She had a black eye. 'How did you get that?' asked the counsellor as if enquiring about a new pair of jeans. 'A geezer walloped me', replied the girl. The counsellor looked very serious and got the girl to tell her the story, which was this:

She had been in a pub and a man whom she knew quite well was making facetious remarks. They started 'needling' each other. The girl then explained that she'd deserved the black eye "cos I'd given him worse than he'd given me' and he only gave her the black eye after she'd 'glassed 'im', meaning that she'd stuck a broken glass in his face for which he needed many stitches. The counsellor smiled and congratulated the girl on sticking up for herself.

This girl had come from an appalling background where she had been beaten by a step-father and possibly sexually abused. It must be obvious that you don't deal with this by encouraging her to become a terrorist. There was another factor in play here too: the notion that young women need to become tough to deal with a nasty world. I've seen far too many teenage girls in the classroom and outside who are being turned into a breed of emotionally ugly and unpleasant women by misguided adults who have confused the words 'assertive' and 'aggressive'.

On another occasion in a different organization a youth worker came in with a 17-year-old girl and her friend. They formed a close, closed circle. There was classical music playing on a radio which they took objection to and the worker eventually said: 'Are they trying to force-feed us a dose of culture?' They were aggressive, and eventually I heard one of the girls say, to loud laughter, 'So I said "piss off I've got better things to do"'. The youth worker replied: 'If he's annoying you why shouldn't you chuck a glass of beer over his head. Good going.'

In the classroom the problems of over-identification with teenagers are also present and manifest themselves in a deeply misguided approach. Again there is a reaction against the 'old school' where children were treated like army recruits and force-fed Latin verbs and trigonometry in grammar schools or sent off to what was considered the failed camp at the Secondary Modern school or 'sec. mod'. Then there was a reaction against the reaction as Kenneth Baker swung into stride to bring the 'old school' back with a vengeance. In order to repair the damage done by regimented schooling (which was not education), some teachers in the name of free speech allowed behaviour in classrooms which was downright anti-social. Pupils were allowed to be disruptive and grew up rude and ignorant of skills they needed in order to make sense and meaning out of being alive. I am talking about the excesses here, not the middle ground of teaching staff who know how to behave in a classroom and are therefore valuable models for pupils to learn about their own behaviour. But unfortunately it is the excessive behaviour, rather than ordinary or usual conduct, which gets people's attention, and the headlines. What this sets up is not only bad for children, but continues something one might call the predictable pendulum, or a reactive chain of events. The pendulum works like this: (1) Teachers over-discipline and treat children like army recruits. (2) The 'other side' calls this outrageous and insists on urgent change. (3) As a reaction to over-disciplining, the pendulum swings to the left, children are then under-disciplined. (4) Bad exam results and outrage from the other side who insist that their way was right all along, and that that woolly-headed liberals have created chaos in schools. (5) Pendulum swings back to the right. (6) Pupil hospitalized from corporal punishment. (7) New educational research shows that old 'evidence' on exam results was wrong. Better exam results gained from more co-operative ways of learning. (8) Pendulum swings back to the left. (9) In social studies girls cut out pictures of naked women and stick men's heads on top... (10) Some labour

councils declare policies on positive images of homosexuality...
(11) Uproar. (12) Pendulum swings back to the right...

When asked, as I was many times, by newspapers for comments about Ealing's and Haringey's decision to make a policy statement about wanting to combat anti-homosexual images through education I said that it had set the cause of sex education back many years. I explained that it was bad enough having to take flak from the Moral Right without finding yourself knee-capped in your own back yard. As an educator my concern is not to have attitudes or anti-attitudes but to introduce pupils to the subject of enquiry which is the area of sexuality and relationships. Of course educators should be aware that there are extreme biases and prejudices in society and should introduce pupils to this knowledge which pupils must then decide about for themselves. If the subjects of sexuality and relationships are being dealt with properly in a classroom homosexuality is part of the spectrum of sexuality and is attended to as such. It may be appropriate to invite in a visiting speaker who is active in homosexual rights, so long as a staff member is present. I stress this latter point because I was most disturbed in one school I visited to find that a staff member was not present during a visit from a person from Gay Rights, who was not a trained teacher. My first concern was that he was only about 20 years old. My second was what he told me he'd said in the classroom. He had made the seemingly innocuous comment: 'Being homosexual is no different from being like anyone else. We're all human beings and we're as normal as anyone else is.' Homosexuality cannot be properly talked about within the realms of opposing adjectives like normal or abnormal. For in one way homosexuality is *not* normal, in that it is not conventional, usual or ordinary. So when questions are asked about whether homosexuality should be 'taught in schools' as being normal or abnormal the questions are impossible to answer. For homosexuality is not for a start 'taught' by anyone who would call themselves an educator. In its context within sex education it is discussed, and in that discussion it will emerge that homosexual people form a minority in society. We might then discuss why we have a history of persecuting all kinds of minorities.

Ealing's and Haringey's decision does not tackle the real problem of there being no curriculum laid down for sex *education* and no teachers properly trained in it. If anyone suggested that anti-Hitler programmes were introduced into schools I hope the scheme would be rejected. There is a subject called history which it is vitally important to place in a moral framework. This subject includes descriptions of mass murders. No-one has yet suggested that pupils are encouraged to commit mass murder because of history lessons. Neither has anyone suggested that young girls are encouraged to anorexia through Byronic poetry. It flies in the face of important educational principles to engage in anti-sexist, anti-racist or anti-heterosexual-bias policies as such. The subjects in themselves (ie sexism, racism, sexual orientation) must be discussed within their larger context and introduced not as dogmatic statements of 'Thou shalt not be sexist', etc. but as areas of important enquiry. Any 'anti' policy is by definition a reaction, and only continues the predictable swing of the pendulum. Education is not concerned with reaction but about solidly based *action*. That action is the delicate one of giving individual children the key to their own minds and hearts and helping them to find out how to use it. If we think we have been ravaged by racist attitudes the long-term answer lies not in programmes of anti-racism but in integrative, sound education. I am already hearing the rumblings that were bound to follow on from anti-racist programmes and that is white pupils complaining of discrimination against whites. This in turn will fuel even more racist feelings and so the reactive chain will go on. This kind of reactive chain, or the pendulum movement I have described, is a macrocosmic version of what a friend calls 'the smack/stroke syndrome'. There cannot be a parent or teacher who doesn't know what this syndrome feels like, even if they haven't actually named it. It arises when you get tense from overwork, worry or whatever, snap or lash out at a child when he or she doesn't really deserve more than a mild rebuke. Then minutes, hours or days later you are suddenly overcome with remorse and 'stroke' the child better. The syndrome is, if you like, the manifestation of unresolved tensions and ambivalences within us, the struggle between our 'better' and 'worse' selves. It is often the discrepancy between the 'good' parent we would like to be and the real person who falls short of this ideal. The smack/stroke syndrome is difficult to cure because most of us were brought up on it. It is in fact a habitually unbalanced state. For the gravitational resting place of the pendulum is in the middle where feelings of conflict are reconciled and where good, solid action takes place. The habitual imbalance, however, the swing from right to left, carries on a reactive chain of events which has no resolution. Children who suffer the smack/stroke syndrome are punished and then spoiled in turn. They are over-punished for something quite small and then spoiled at a time when they might be being quite unpleasant and could do with a sharp word. They are then further punished to compensate for the spoiling and further spoiled to compensate for the punishment. It is nothing if not a messy, exasperating business.

A parent who found that she was in this syndrome, but got out of it when she saw what was happening, described her experience:

I was ratty one minute, then guilty for being ratty the next, and then I got ratty again for being such a wimp as to feel guilty. I talked it over with Chris [her husband] and realized I was going from one extreme to the other and the poor kids mustn't have known where they were half the time. It took a little while after realizing it was going on for me to stop it. I can't say exactly how it happened, but I'd obviously been thinking about it. Chris and I had been away for a weekend on our own to have some time away from the kids. It ended up with me bursting into tears and saying what an awful mother I was. But I felt better and stronger and then just bided my time. Then one morning I just got up and said: 'This is it. If I want to stop I'd better start now.' I went downstairs earlier than usual and when the children came down I was ready for them. First of all I said 'Good morning' in a rather over-firm, over-cheerful voice. But I'd said it properly. Usually I said a mumbled 'morning' with my back turned to them as I washed the dishes from the night before. This time I faced them. They knew something was up. Their faces were a mixture of pleasant surprise and extreme wariness. Part of them was wondering what the hell was coming next and was not sure if they were going to like it.

I got them their breakfasts more slowly than usual and sat down with them while they ate, another thing I tended not to do because I was usually doing something else. By the time they went to school I was feeling a great deal stronger, although also as if I was in some kind of daze, as if someone else was doing this not me. But I carried on. When the children were around I spoke more slowly than usual, and took a deep breath when I felt like snapping. When you ask me what I did that's the only way I can describe it. Something in me decided I was tired of being pushed back and forth between irritation and guilt. I didn't read any books to find the answer. Maybe I decided that if I didn't get irritated, or act irritated in the first place, then I wouldn't get guilty. So I developed this for a while, for myself. If something went wrong I dealt with it calmly, and the children soon got the message. Paul, the eldest, came up to me after a few days and said: 'There's something got into you, Mum. You're different'. I told him I intended to stay that way — and I have.

Chris, Anne's husband, said that from his point of view the change in Anne and the children was considerable:

> We agreed that because I have a far higher salary than Anne I should continue full-time work after the children were born, and Anne would resume part-time work after they went to school. So Anne had been the person who has been with them most. I noticed she was getting very irritable and that everything seemed too much for her, even if I took the children away for hours on end. It was the weekend away which changed it all. We walked and talked a great deal. She began to unwind and on the last day she cried her heart out and said something like: 'I can see it now. I let them wind me up, then I explode, then I feel guilty and get down in the dumps. I'm a lousy mother.' I reminded her that they were both our children, and that if things were going wrong it was my fault too. We discussed us both getting up earlier for a while to get a proper grip of the day before the kids came down. And we've stuck to that. It's meant getting to bed earlier and missing out on some of the evening. But the kids are eleven and nine now, so that won't have to go on for much longer. Anne's much calmer altogether and the children are calmer and happier too. It's made a hell of a lot of difference to us all.

The difference it would make to education and to society if this smack/stroke syndrome and the pendulum effect it causes and aggravates were slowly stopped would be beyond measurement. The best of educational philosophy and tradition would be blended in with the best in modern thinking and facilities to provide for children and all the adults who are involved with them a qualitative improvement in lives. The quantitative and predictably mechanical push of the pendulum to left or right takes up a considerable amount of energy, and this would also be saved for better purposes.

In the classroom the swinging pendulum ensures that it is indoctrination and not education which is taking place. Strangely enough it produces the old kind of 'moral' teaching-on-the-blackboard regime. Only this time the commandments are different and read: 'Thou shalt not be sexist; thou shalt not be racist.' I've not had pupils query anti-sexist classes, except when a boy said, as a huge complaint, that girls could be sexist too. I said of course they could, and often were, and hadn't this been discussed? He claimed not, although he might well have been mistaken. My problem with some anti-sexist programmes is that they've been just that, programmes. I have often heard young people repeat them parrot fashion to me without *personal* conviction of their truth and without having transformed the knowledge so that it's theirs and can therefore be used for their personal development. A 16-year-old boy said to me recently in a classroom: 'Women should have equal rights.' He said it blandly and without personal conviction. So I asked mildly: 'Should they? Why do you think they, we, should?' 'Because they've been put down. and because they deserve a chance — and because they're people, just like men,' he replied. 'Why do *you* think women should have equality?' I said. 'He's just repeating what we learned in general studies,' said another boy, while the first boy wondered how to answer. 'What generally do you think about this question of "equal rights"?' I asked, opening to up the whole group. There was an awkward silence broken by one of the girls saying that it was only right that women had equality. I nodded. 'Can we talk about something more interesting, Miss?' asked one of the boys politely.

At the end of the day we want either intelligent, open, affectionate individuals, or closed, programmed people knowing only rules and regulations. If we want the former then educational principles must not be swept overboard by gales blowing from the Moral Right, or the Moral Left.

CHAPTER ELEVEN

Cowboys and Indians

My own work with young people is done because I enjoy it and am rewarded by it. It is also a kind of investment. Unlike market investments however, I will have to accept the 'return' on my work as being unquantifiable. How can you quantify the feeling when a young woman stops you in the street and says: 'Hallo, Miss. Do you remember me? You came to our school when I was in the fifth year...?' I am warmed and what I can only describe as 'added to' by these encounters. On one occassion one of them *was* measurable. I had left a dinner party at about midnight and was walking back to the car parked some distance away. I came to a house throbbing with pop music and the loud voices of young people. As I passed, three or four boys or young men came spilling out of the door and started making suggestive remarks to me. I thought they were probably harmless, but because it was late and there was a number of them I was on my guard too. I carried on walking and they followed me down the road and caught up with me. At this stage I felt increasing alarm, but tried to act calmly. So I turned to face them and was going to tell them rather severely that chasing a woman down the road was threatening, that they ought to know this and shouldn't do it. As I opened my mouth to speak the teenager who had got to me first stopped in horror, 'Oh no', he said in absolute dismay, 'it's Miss.'

I have been grateful many times for being 'Miss', mainly because this exacting and privileged position has given me insight into understanding teenagers. I stand sometimes alone in finding this age group endearing, surprising, funny and, given the opportunities, capable of far more kindness, devotion and serious commitment than people credit them with. I find the humour of teenagers has saved me from potenially embarrassing situations and that they have not condemned me for the mistakes I have made. On the contrary, my own honesty in admitting when I am mistaken has produced from both male and female pupils a corresponding protective impulse. As a girl said once when I apologized for giving a less than clear description of the 'safe period', 'Don't worry, Miss. Compared to my mum talking about it you are a star.' I may have aspired to greater things than being a star at explaining 'natural family planning' but I couldn't think of any of them right at that moment.

Since much of my work has been with young people who have problems I am also aware of the aggression and menace which some teenagers present. Some teenagers set out to be menacing, and when they happen to be physically powerful boys they acheive their intention. Many times in the street, although not in the classroom, I have felt menaced by youths who set out to be intimidating and threatening. And I have been more fortunate than many in not having suffered, so far, any actual physical damage. The classroom is the only place I know of where this kind of person can be offered a real opportunity to change. Yet, as I have already stated, this opportunity has not been taken up in a serious and committed enough way. By the time boys who have not learned about self-respect at home are spilling out of school gates at the age of 16, much of the damage has already been done, and once they are on the streets it is much more difficult to reach out and help them.

There is also nowadays a menace coming from a certain kind of teenage girl. In the confusion caused by losing sight of what real education is, this girl has been taught something called her 'rights'. Unfortunately in indoctrinating her with her rights people forgot to inform her of her responsibilities, and the two should be inseparable. At a time of rising figures on child abuse and incest it is important for teenagers to know what rights they have, both civil and legal. It is a natural concomitant of this for them to know what rights other people have and therefore what responsiblities everyone has to help ensure the continuing existence of human rights *for everyone*. When teenagers tell me in school that they have been learning their rights I am therefore not always as pleased as I might be, considering that I argue childrens' causes. I am depressed that for some the alternative to young people being abused is seen as arming children in a way which causes them to be abusive. What is so distressing is that the way to get it right is not difficult. It is not as if one were asking for impossibly complex things to happen, but for things quite simple and staightforward. A little while ago I was asked to be a consultant, one of many, on a book for young teenagers. The people putting the book together were extremely concerned to get it right and went to great lengths and considerable expense to do this. I thought, and still do think, that their efforts were admirable. When the final version of the manuscript came through to me it contained a section on abuse of young people. It had in it under this section the following sentence: 'It is better to be suspicious and over-cautious *as a way of life* (my italic) than to fall victim of an attacker.'

I had spent a good deal of time before getting this manuscript talking with various people about incest, and the work with young people which has begun in this area. I said that as long as the work was done in context it was a much-needed addition to young peoples lives. When asked what I meant, I explained that since the ability to trust is one of the most fragile and important of human qualities, and an ability without which good relationships of any kind cannot happen, I hoped that this was never lost sight of. In other words if young children were helped to be more alert to danger without jeopardising their ability to trust, that was fine. I also explained that young children *do* trust, and this is a great part of their appeal — for most of us want, despite difficulties, to be trustworthy. I have been pushed on this point a number of times because people haven't seen clearly what I have meant. What I have been trying to get at is that the symbiotic relationship between adult and child is one where the young child is perforce dependant on us. The child therefore trusts that because he or she has to have the hope of growing, we will deliver the goods. When we do, the young child or baby trusts more. Although delivering the goods is sometimes extremely hard work for an adult, the child's display of trust is one of the crucial factors in making the effort worthwhile, and the relationship then grows and strengthens. By the time most children learn that we are not always trustworthy they are old enough to know, safely, that we are as imperfect as they are and that this is all right. The point is that the quality of trust is a part of a whole picture, and that children need to learn to be cautious *within the context of keeping intact their ability to trust.* It would be a tragedy of ghastly proportions if a generation of children growing up now had their ability to trust impaired by an over-stressed or wrongly-empha-sized need to be cautious. There is another way of writing the sentence sent to me to achieve what is needed and I wrote this: 'While it is a very important part of your life to learn to love and trust you also need to learn to be cautious'.

What really alarmed me about the proposed sentence is that three other consultants, all experts in the area of child abuse, had passed it without demur. It would have gone into the book as written to be read by thousands and maybe hundreds of thousands of young people. The sentence illustrates once more the dangers of reactive behaviour, which can only ever cause damage in the long term, and sometimes in the short term as well. 'It is better to be suspicious and over-cautious as a way of life...': such a horrific formula, as well as being a death sentence to vitality and full humanity, is primarily a reaction to the horrors of child abuse. The long-term effects of people being constantly suspicious are not difficult to forsee. They will bring about less love, more unhappiness and more violence. They might then in the long term produce the utterly absurd state of affairs where children are re-deified from our reactive need for purity, innocence and trust. In turn that will produce, as it must, a further wave of child abuse from a generation of parents unused to these qualities and therefore unable to deal with them.

Attitudes on the right and left of the pendular swing take many different forms, and, as Sarah Kennedy said on a daytime show for Thames Television, 'The one person I wouldn't like to be these days is a child.' She made this comment after a Conservative MP had talked about the sanctity of the family and parents' rights, a Labour politician had talked about the reality of children's lives, a studio audience had shown how petrified they were of homosexuality and I had tried to explain what sex education actually is. Since that time I've drawn verbal sketches of parents I've met on the right and left of the political spectrum, and what is perhaps *not* surprising is that some of the sketches are almost identical. There is the (conservative) father who says it is his job to protect his child from the evils of the wicked world. As a businessman he is ruthless, and aware somewhere at the back of his mind that he has 'got on' by being precisely this. He has cheated and been dishonest, and although he wouldn't actually say this out loud he knows it. He is therefore determined that his children do not lie and cheat. He will provide the very best for them in terms of private schools, private tuition, education facilities and will give them everything money can buy. He wants his children to be educated, and also 'moral'. He may have been immoral himself to get a good secure base, but who wouldn't, he thinks, given half a chance? This man splits his life into two camps, the big bad world of business and the world of his home and offspring. He would almost kill to keep his children from his own 'real adult world' which he perceives as treacherous. His children are different from this. They are 'other'. This man doesn't know it but he wants a miracle. That is his deepest hope. The miracle he wants is that his children will not see this split; that they will not question his daytime self, but will accept as gospel only what he wants to tell them. The other miracle he wants is that by his children's doing this, he will be absolved, his actions vindicated. They will, in other words, make his own treacheries worth it. They will redeem him. When his children utterly defeat him by being ordinary, normal kids he is dejected and wonders angrily why they wouldn't just accept what he had to offer. Why did they have to spoil things? He wonders, among other things, what *he* did to deserve this.

There is the woman on the left of the political spectrum. She has worked throughout her children's lives taking advantage of creches and the kind of childcare facilities she has fought hard to get. She is a media woman, and has had to kick and fight to get on in a man's world. She was badly discriminated against in the early stages of her career. This went towards making her ruthless. Luckily both her children were daughters (her comment, not mine) and she dotes on them. In the office she lies and cheats without even thinking about it because that's what you do. The end justifies the means. At home she is positively delighted that her two teenage offspring are growing up in an environment she helped to create where discrimination has become a dirty word. She is proud that they will have an easier time of it than she did. To meet her at home and at work is to experience moral schizophrenia: the day time bully and the night time softie, the manipulator and the craven woman. I say 'craven' because her daughters are like goddesses to her, her own work and hope incarnate. Sometimes a wistful look comes into this woman's eyes. She wants, without knowing it, her daughters to make her own treacheries worthwhile. She wants them to redeem her lost values. And, of course, they won't.

The old saying that children break their parents' hearts has some of this in it, making live the cliché that 'truth will out'. For if in truth we need them to do better than us to *repair* what we have done wrong, to rescue our stranded hopes and selves, then give them an impossible and offensive burden both personally and generally. On a personal level they are visited by our ghosts, by the need to do unspecified strange things for us for our own sakes, so they are not free. On a general level they are hemmed in by many of our nightmares made concrete, like acid rain and nuclear stock piles. It will be their task to divest themselves of the former, sometimes brutally, and to sort out the latter so that *their* children come into a world worth living in.

Parents break childrens' hearts too. I went to a recreational centre once to write an article about childrens' holidays and to see whether what was being offered was genuine and generous and not mean-spirited. In fact the organizers, the workers, and the centre itself were all of a very high standard. This particular holiday was in a beatiful part of the Wye Valley, and the children had forest, river-bank, hedgerow and a private swimming pool to explore and make use of. The workers went to endless trouble to make sure their young charges were happy, and also learning. There were games, adventures, musical evenings, plays, sing-songs and plenty of affection for the odd occasion when a little one had time to remember to miss home.

In the middle of the week it was a boy's birthday. He had been on these holidays before, and was to be nine. One of the workers came down in the evening and said wearily: 'We're going to have to do something about Pete again.' Pete's parents had apparently ditched him as they were wont to do. They seemed to have plenty of money, yet Pete arrived in scruffy clothes and shoes. He got out of their large, very expensive car always looking pale and tired. All the half-dozen workers got together and made some cards and wrapped a few small presents. The following morning at breakfast they called for attention for the announcement of Pete's birthday, and everyone sang 'Happy Birthday' to him. He looked even more strained than usual. That morning he loitered around the hallway waiting for the postman to come. No birthday card arrived.

At times like that you can't take on a child's suffering, not unless he or she asks you to. You can only watch for the smallest sign that you're wanted and be ready to give. We carried on with the day ostensibly treating Pete like anyone else, while being alert to any signal from him. None came. That night we felt mute with pain and impotence.

In the sea of bidden and unbidden faces which come into memory in writing about children, Pete's is there, a wraith to remind us that he too has a place in all this. And if children must own what they know the burden of ownership is heavy for some. More than a few of the children you meet in classrooms come to school each day with hurts of this kind, and because of our growing awareness of the needs of children and the culpability of adults, it is easy to react in horror and therefore make worse what is already bad. One cannot 'cane' parents who forgot their only child's ninth birthday, and would it help the child if we could? This is why it is the purpose of education not to be reactive. Schools are supposed to provide a broad, balanced and un-hysterical education for all children, and within this encompass carefully the needs of the children whose parents haven't known best. Any work on sexuality, child abuse, racism, needs therefore to be carefully looked at to make sure that it is conducted within a framework of sound educational principles. It must not be carried out from political expediency or pressing social needs unless the subject is first placed in context and conducted as part of a wider pattern of learning.

What all the conflict surrounding sex education actually shows is that it is becoming more and more important for people to have the ability to use their judgement. For if in the mass of figures, conflicting facts, stories and politicking, ordinary people could not use their common sense to 'cut through the cackle' we would really be in even more trouble. In a multi-faceted society where the media slings statistics and 'information' at us, it largely depends upon which publication you read as to which 'facts' you get. The only way for people to know what is right is for them to be educated to have the ability to discern, and to decide for them-selves. Indoctrination of any kind militates against a person's thinking abilities and therefore against his or her developing the ability to form sound judgements. If there is one quality school could be giving young people that would be of immeasureable value, it is the ability to think clearly and therefore to judge wisely. The most important ability the home can nurture is the ability to love, surely the most difficult and rewarding ability of all.

Some parents say that they find teenagers more difficult to love than when they were small children, perhaps because it is not always easy to see that love is as much concerned with what you *don't* do as with what you *do*. It shows itself as much in the difficult standing back and not interfering as it does in the moving forward to offer help. And teenagers are at the difficult time of moving away from wanting a certain kind of love from parents towards being ready and able to give special love to one other person. They are in between the tail end of still needing to be held by us, and the beginning of adult love of their own which will invlove their holding someone else. It may be because they are in this vulnerable position that we continue driving, herding them through the narrowing gap of political and financial expediency. At either side of the gap, to the right and left of it, stand two groups of people each determined either that those young people should go *their* way or that they should not go the way of the people standing opposite. If the picture formed by this looks like something from an old-fashioned Western with thousands of head of steer being driven towards a narrow gorge while the goodies and baddies turn them first this way and then that, then it's pretty near what I'm trying to describe. When you realize further that the goodies of the old films, the cowboys, are now the baddies because we now know that the American Indians were in fact the victims of the white man, not his aggressor, then the analogy becomes more and more interesting. In this context the cowboys are in my opinion on the right hand side of the gorge. They are the people who think they have a right to call morality their own, and it is perhaps in reaction to this that the people on the left hand side have committed their own errors. The people on the right hand side of the gorge don't view it this way of course. They have said for years that the nasty Indians are baddies intent on collecting scalps and indulging in wicked, pagan festivals.

I have thought a great deal about the adults standing at the head of that gorge, and even more about the thousands of children who are herded through it. I can only imagine that the adults on the right suffer from a form of paranoia which means that they must view everyone who does not agree with their point of view as dangerous. Which is why they have tried to make Indians out of the rest of us and suggest that we are rooted educationally in paganism and degeneracy. Their views are not therefore so much sincerely held as fanatically so — a condition of which as a result of suffering it themselves they accuse their opponents. (Thus the headlines featured earlier about Loony Left schools and naked women.) Any sign of independent life is seen as a danger that they can't cope with, which is why the full spectrum of human nature with all its attendant complexities frightens them. It is some kind of primeval fright where the dread of the beast of chaos coming crashing through the undergrowth would make every man and woman of them retreat to the security and order of a well-defended symmetrical nuclear bunker. For in the attitudes which prevail it is interesting that these people rage against sex outside marriage and support a nuclear defence policy. What further distresses me about such people is that they have hijacked the words 'morality' and 'decency' and taken them away from common behaviour. The rest of us they then proclaim immoral and indecent because we do not have what they have stolen from us. It is all very tortuous. They have tried to hijack love itself and put it up for a terrible ransom which the rest of us cannot pay because we are not their version of God-fearing, law-abiding citizens. They have dressed themselves in the cloths of modesty but in fact they are wolves of a kind. They certainly devour children, and through doing so haunt us from generation to generation. Because some people do not recognize wolves dressed up in decent clothing, the latter sometimes have the ear of those in high places, and much as I am against violence we might insist that the ears of people in high places are regularly syringed. That way those in high places who are wolves themselves might find that the voices of the rest of us become too loud for them to continue to pretend they cannot hear us. Meanwhile, the people on the left of the gorge have reacted against having their clothes stolen. They too have taken up cudgels. I didn't enjoy meeting the young woman who mindlessly berated me for not being working class and being therefore 'an oppressor'. The unsure, vulnerable person behind this rhetoric was not any easier to meet.

While all this goes on one of the biggest moral issues affecting young people and the rest of us continues relatively unabated. The problem of consumerism and its worrying ethics has powerful effects on young people's lives. For a start, the consumer market, for its own profit, has commodified youth and made being young into its own triumph, into a thing apart. In a way, therefore, the market place has ripped up generational connections at both ends. In increasing the generation gap from our end it has made sure that fad, fashion and phase have such a high turnover that only people with the energy of 16-year-olds can keep up. This distances *us*. By making youth into a thing apart, into its own glory, it also distances *them*. This has the effect of making maturity something to be avoided rather than cherished, for maturity is seen as a dissapointment after the 'hype' of being young.

A good many young people who initially claim they prefer the television or video to adult company are products, and victims, of this pressure. They soon become prey to an isolation which they cannot articulate. This means they need *more* human time spent with them, not less, for despite appearances to the contrary they need more reassurance that we are still there, and there for *them*. A mother in her thirties made her own discovery of this when, following the break-up with her husband, she reclaimed her son from the video:

> After Michael left, Alan became very withdrawn. All he wanted
> to do was to be alone and watch the video. I let him for a while
> because I thought it might be a kind of mindless consolation for
> him and because I thought perhaps he needed to be away from

me for a bit. I didn't know how much he was blaming me and whether or not he wanted me to break his silence. After a few weeks I decided to restrict the video time and also to make sure that we had meals sitting down together at the table. It was awkward to begin with. It's frightening to realize how soon you lose contact. After a few more weeks of awkwardness he came bounding in from school one day and said: 'Can we go to the Science Museum, Mum? I want to see the models there.' I resisted the urge to sweep him up and hug him and instead took a deep breath and suggested we had tea on the way. As I watched him hopping and skipping along the pavement and brushing against hedges I felt very grateful for his return. After that he began asking me questions about our break-up, Michael's and mine, and I answered them as best I could. One evening we were sitting down over tea and he said: 'Do you have dreams, Mum?' I was so startled. I was almost speechless. I said 'Yes', I did, and we started talking about dreams. It became a one-removed way of talking about Michael and after a few months it served its purpose and the 'dream-talk' stopped. But sometimes if he's a bit tired or clingy he'll still say 'Remember the dreams, Mum', and I give him an extra big hug. It occurs to me that children don't know we have dreams unless we tell them. Perhaps they think it's something only children have.

'Being there' for young people is in fact a moral issue in itself, as well as an educational one. This young woman discovered for herself, for instance, the truth that many children don't believe we have dreams any more because we don't pass important ones on to them, probably because we think they don't want to hear them. But since the telling of dreams either in symbolic or actual form is an important link between generations, the living dreams and nightmares are so much more important to attend to than the celluloid ones which the personal computer can project. For what is the worth of human emotions? How does this compare with computer teaching? Many of the moral issues which surround education and young people are as complex as the world in which schools, children and parents exist. They are as complex as knowing that presidents lie, as do prime ministers, and that government officials are economical with the truth. They are as complex as knowing that wars are devastating and that the people who order them are usually heads of government who want children to be good little boys and girls and teenagers to obey the forces of law and order. What alarms me is not that young people may stumble across any of these contradictions, but that they might not. Because on their ability to get a better grasp of moral issues than we have rests the main hope of repair and re-building.

Fundamental to real moral education is a search for personal truth. It offers also the essential encouragement towards the realization that life is worth living in its entirety, and that it is an obscenity to want only the 'good bits' of it. The pleasure principle has replaced the search for joy and meaning and is in itself pornographic, for it is partial in that it does not tell the whole truth. I have found young people to be fascinated by discussions of difference between pleasure and joy. They have engaged whole-heartedly in discussions of cause and effect and the difference between short-term profit and long-term gain. They have shown themselves to be tired of sex being the whipping post of moral standards, and of moral values resting in girls rather than in both sexes. Young people have shown time and again that they want a general education in morality, sexuality and relationship.

So what is to be done? At the moment the International Planned Parenthood Federation (IPPF) is in the process of looking at the political management of sex education both in Britain and in Europe. Dr Philip Meredith, Programme Adviser, and Alan Beattie of the Institute of Education are aiming to draw a picture of the political dimension of the subject through interviews conducted here and in other European countries. Through interviewing a cross-section of people who are involved with sex education they should be able to give us an idea of who the influential interest groups are and make critical recommendations.

Meanwhile, the Policy Studies Institute (PSI) has already conducted, as discussed earlier, a major study of teenagers' and parents' attitudes to sex education from interviewing over 400 people in three major British cities. Isobel Allen's findings, *Education in Sex and Personal Relationships,* were published in February 1987. At the Press Conference to launch this report, Ms Allen said:

The last major study on sex education was done 10 years ago. In 1974 Christine Farrell published her research which showed that 96 per cent of parents wanted sex education to take place in schools. My own research has come up with the same figure more than 10 years later. Therefore the debate about whether sex education should take place in schools has been whipped up out of all proportion. Very few parents told me they didn't want the subject done in schools.

She went on to say:

> Parents told us horrific stories about their own lack of sex educa-
> tion, and this is one of the reasons they want their children to
> have better information than they did. Parents don't want their
> children to catch AIDS, to have unwanted pregnancies or broken
> marriages, and many of them said that they wanted their children
> to have a realistic rather than a rosy view of the opposite sex. The
> teenagers themselves confirmed this when they said that school
> discussions in a group were very often their only opportunity to
> listen to how people of the opposite sex felt about things. The
> boys especially said this. Boys were very concerned that they might
> be missing something because they were told so little about girls.

Isobel Allen's report makes the following recommendations:

> It should be the aim of all secondary schools to follow the pattern
> established in certain local authorities and schools of integrating
> sex education into a programme of personal and social education
> for *all* pupils, *both boys and girls*. (My italic.)
> Schools should make as much use as possible of films, television
> programmes, videos and other visual presentation. These were
> much appreciated by school children.
> Class discussions under the guidance of a teacher should be
> encouraged and extended. Teenagers found discussions of this
> kind particularly helpful in relating facts to relationships. *They
> stressed the value of learning from others through hearing a variety
> of views.* (My italic.)
> The use of expert and sensitive outsiders giving talks or leading
> discussions at schools should be encouraged. Both parents and
> teenagers were in favour of 'outsiders' as long as they were clearly
> identified and had particular expertise.
> Schools should regard it as an important part of their role to
> correct the influence of pornographic videos and magazines *which
> were thought to have a particularly damaging effect on boys*. (My
> italic.)
> *Priority should be given to training teachers in the skills needed
> to handle these topics* in the classroom and when they are
> approached informally by teenagers. (My italic.)

I would add to this only that the *way* of training these teachers
be considered extremely carefully. My own recommendations
would be that training should ensure:

(a) That the difference between subjectivity and objectivity is
fully understood.

(b) That the difference between education and indoctrination is similarly understood.
(c) That the boundaries of personal disclosure, particularly with younger pupils, are handled extremely carefully.

I would suggest that sex education has been 'up for grabs' for far too long. Like Isobel Allen I too think that the debate on sex education has been whipped up in the face of overwhelming evidence that parents want this subject to be taught in schools, and wanted this consistently for more than a decade. Why, in the face of this, has the Moral Right been allowed to get away with claiming that parents do not want this subject taught? What power is invested in them that they may do this? Sex education has been prone to media meddling and political interference of a most unhealthy kind, the kind that ignores real public opinion. It often appears as though anyone with power or influence can take over running of this subject while the people who are actually involved in it — pupils, parents and teachers — are forced to take a back seat. Teachers need to be trained, and the institutes which train teachers need a mandate to do so and a programme to work with. As part of this, books for pupils in particular need to be produced which are compiled by people working in this field and which have a wide reference base. Until this happens spurious arguments will hold sway.

At the moment, children in the developed world are nailed to a form of political expediency which appears to suggest that the introduction of young people to the ability to use their own judgement is tantamount to riotous assembly. While this stalling goes on, bad politics make young people biddable and ignorance makes them both angry and forlorn. I once made up a list, based on reading an article about the 'offences' of sex education. I tried to look at what is *really* offensive in the classroom, or at least to explore this. The list emerged in the form of a number of questions which went like this:

Is it offensive to presume:
—that every child in the classroom is English?
—that every child is European?
—that every child is white?
—that every child has two parents?
—that every child has been well taken care of?
—that every child knows what love is?
—that every child is a sexual being?
—that every child has brothers and/or sisters?

—that every child was wanted?
—that every child is well fed?
—that every child has the same needs?

The only thing it is not 'offensive' to presume here is that every child is a sexual being. Every other assumption is incorrect, if nothing else, and worrying enough for that. Yet the Moral Right is now suggesting that basic biology is all that is needed. This is blind stupidity in the light of bringing up children in a highly complicated world. What the classroom can offer young people is work between groups and individuals carried out skilfully so that pupils learn from each other and through their personal development how to become more themselves. In this endeavour there is no room for 'moral policing' by the right or the left. A child will only contribute uniquely to society if giving the opportunity to be unique — allowed to have a mind and heart of his or her own. This will only occur if children are encouraged to think for themselves *against the day when they will have to*. If we believe there are too many teenagers who behave mindlessly it is because we have failed individually and collectively to enable them to achieve what possible. A 'moral guard' of a new or old order is superfluous in rectifying this, for education is not about indoctrination or inculcation. In the end it's about love; it's about difficult times and the sharing of difficulties. And it's about whether we're big enough people to accommodate the reality that our hopes are our own and that other people's minds are not our property. I do not think any child's bundle of circumstances, fantasies, dreams and disappointments should be 'policed'. I think it should be respected as belonging to that child, who is like no other and who shares, and needs to find, much in common with us all.

First love, first sex

A practical guide to relationships

First love, first sex is a book for today's young people. It explores how early sexual relationships begin, develop and sometimes end; how sex and love can fit together and flourish. Written in conjunction with the Family Planning Association, it offers sound, practical advice on how to fulfil emotional and physical needs, cope with social pressures, sexual problems, and personal responsibilities. *First love, first sex* is a down-to-earth guide to successful relationships.

- Feeling shy and lonely? *First love, first sex* provides an action plan for change.

- Finding it difficult to form satisfying relationships? *First love, first sex* looks at ways of making out.

- Feeling used and angry? *First love, first sex* shows you how to banish self-destructive emotions.

Kaye Wellings is a researcher/writer who has written many articles on a wide range of social and health issues, especially teenage sexuality and pregnancy, for both popular and professional publications. She has contributed to the writing and teaching of several Open University courses and is currently working as Research Officer at the Family Planning Association.

Growing pains

What to do when your children turn into teenagers

As any parent knows, teenagers dominate the telephone, play unbearably loud music, never tidy their rooms, stay out late and are incredibly moody. Despite these frustrations, parents really do care about their kids, are confused about what is happening and don't know what to do.

Growing Pains gives parents the answers they've been crying out for. Dr David Bennett, head of the Adolescent Medical Unit at the Royal Alexandra Hospital for Children in Sydney, Australia, who has three teenagers of his own, explains what makes teenagers behave the way they do and what parents can do to help their kids, and themselves, through the experience.

The author covers every possible issue that parents of adolescents are likely to be confronted with: puberty; behaviour; sexuality; school; the quality of their own marriage and the effect this has on the kids; teenagers and older relations and younger brothers and sisters; specific relationships within the family; diet and problems with diet, such as anorexia nervosa; hygiene; fitness; health; emotional pressures; avoiding dangerous risks, such as drugs; work; letting go.

Dr David Bennett is head of the Adolescent Medical Unit of the Royal Alexandra Hospital for Children in Sydney, which he founded in 1977. He is also a consultant with the World Health Organization, a leading member for the Australian Association for Adolescent Health and one of the principal organizers of the Fourth International Symposium on Adolescent Health.